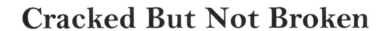

Cracked But Not Broken

Cracked But Not Broken

A COLLECTION OF RECIPES AND LESSONS
FOR PERSONAL GROWTH

SHANNON BURRS

XULON PRESS

Xulon Press
2301 Lucien Way #415
Maitland, FL 32751
407.339.4217
www.xulonpress.com

Cracked But Not Broken
A Collection of Recipes and Life Experiences Toward Personal Growth

Recipe photos throughout book provided by Shannon Burrs.

Lifestyle photos provided by Krista Brinkmeier Photography.

Paperback ISBN-13: 978-1-6628-5937-3
Hard Cover ISBN-13: 978-1-6628-5938-0
Ebook ISBN-13: 978-1-6628-5939-7

Dedication

I would like to dedicate this book to my dad who always made me laugh and feel loved in his short time here on earth. I miss him more than words can say and look forward to the day we meet again.

To my family – thank you for your constant love and never-ending support.

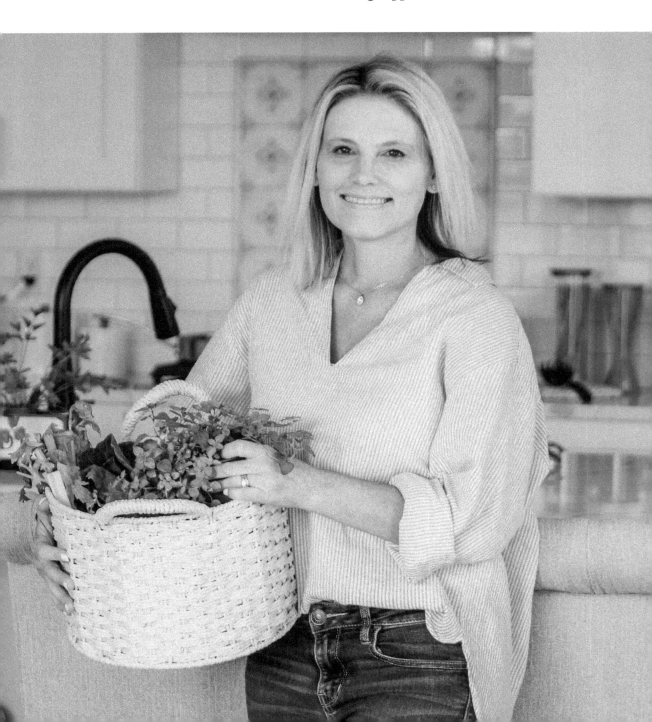

About the Author

SHANNON IS AN AMERICAN COOKBOOK AUTHOR, FOOD blogger and podcast host. She is a Wisconsin native and a Midwest girl with a love for all things wine, cheese, and dairy. Shannon began her career in dentistry as a Registered Dental Hygienist and later discovered a passion for food blogging and writing amidst the Covid Pandemic. She published her first book *A Healthy Balance: In Life and In the Kitchen* in 2021.

After losing her dad to depression, Shannon has devoted much of her time to raising awareness about mental health issues and trying to help eliminate the stigma. This book is just another way to reach people and offer hope for a better tomorrow.

Shannon is married to her husband Brad, and together they have four kids. They are settling into their new farmhouse, and enjoying what life has to offer in the country.

Follow Shannon on her blog and social media for daily inspiration, recipes and farm life. www.faithfoodfarm.com

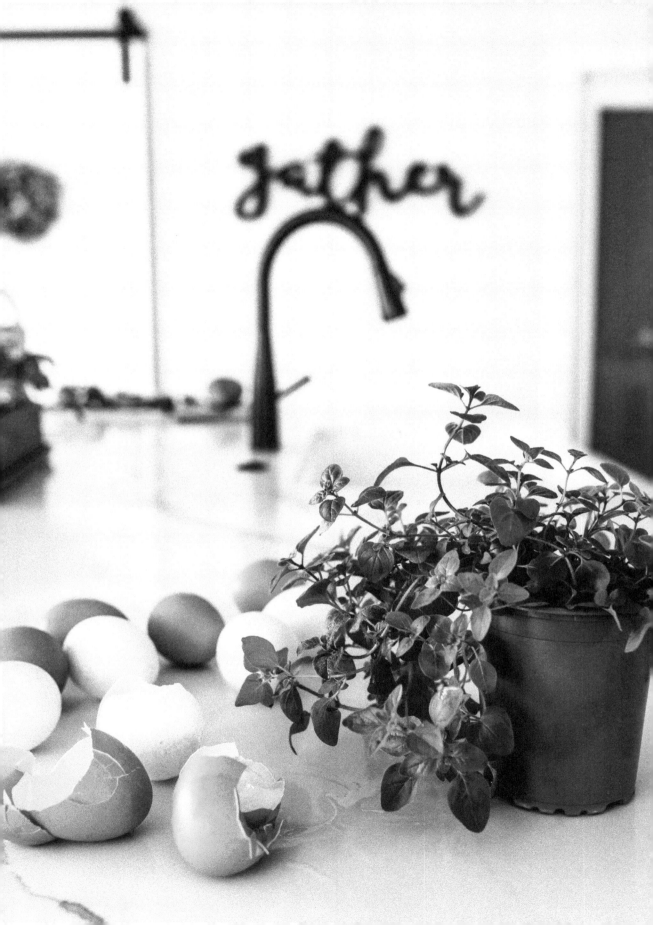

Welcome to My Kitchen

I N MY FIRST BOOK, *A HEALTHY BALANCE: IN LIFE AND IN the Kitchen*, each section included daily reminders for reflection with steps toward self-development. In this book, I want to dig a bit deeper by recognizing some of the harder things we go through in life. Just as recipes need a few more ingredients to achieve their deep, rich flavor, life's hardships leave us with stronger, richer characters.

Over the past two years, I have taken on new ventures of blogging and podcasting since the world around me has expanded. With each new person I meet and talk with, I learn how our life journeys are not as unique as I once thought. We all share similar experiences, feelings, and needs. Each of us are traveling different roads with different obstacles, yet sharing many things in common. We long for our lives to be filled with uncomplicated simplicity, but unfortunately, life is not that predictable.

Our lives can quickly change in the blink of an eye. The more people we meet and places we go, the more we find that life is filled with unknowns–some of it good, some of it not so good.

As a child, I remember having an image of what my life was going to look like. How many kids I was going to have, what kind of job I was going to work and so on. I had my entire life planned out before I was old enough to drive. What I didn't do was plan for heartbreak, divorce, death of a parent or any of the other hardships that would come. These life situations interrupted and *cracked* my plan.

Though we don't like it, life throws us into situations that can leave us feeling hurt and betrayed with heavy hearts. Throughout this book, we'll be talking about how all the cracks in our lives–the good, the bad, and the ugly–shape us.

While we normally shy away from these cracks, I want this book to be a reminder of hope. A reminder that one small crack does not define our lives or leave us broken. Instead, our cracks shape us into the people we are becoming and offer us an opportunity for growth.

"One small crack does not mean you are broken; it means you were put to the test and you didn't fall apart."–**Linda Poindexter**[1]

Table of Contents

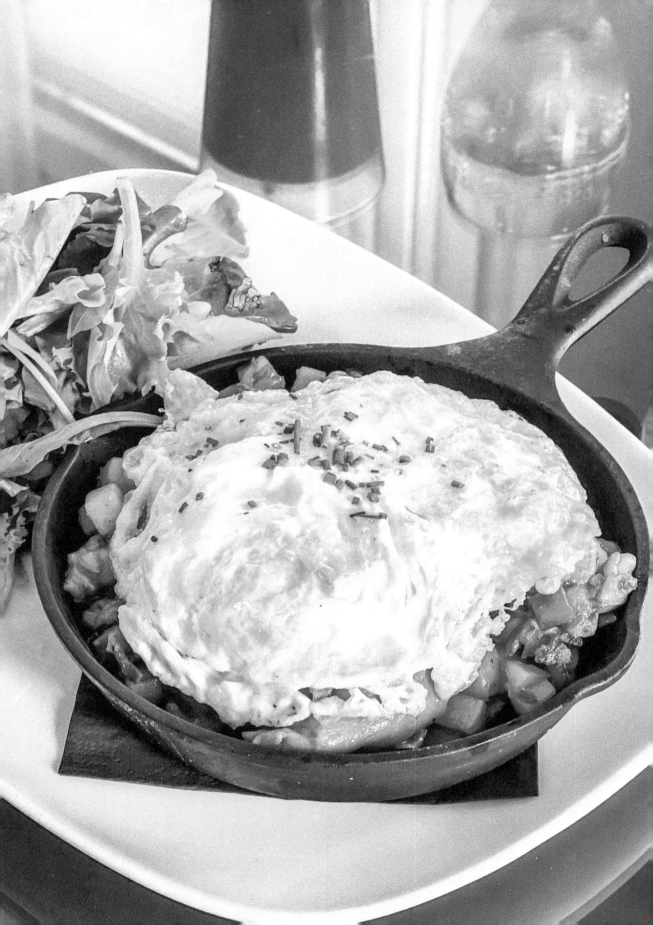

1

Fried from Perfection

"There is no perfection, only beautiful versions of brokenness."
– Shannon L. Alder[2]

WRITING AND PUBLISHING MY FIRST BOOK WAS A LOT OF fun, but it also took a lot of courage to be seen in such a vulnerable way. When I finally held a copy in my hands, many emotions ran through me. As I looked through the pages, I couldn't help but dissect and find all the little things that made it less than perfect. Rather than be proud of my accomplishment, I found all of the ways I could have done it better.

Why do we do this to ourselves?

Here I am again, writing another book about all of the ways our lives are imperfect. The mistakes, misfortunes, the bad stuff that happens to us–the things that really crack our shells.

The hard truth is that not all things go the way we want or expect them to. Whether it be losing a loved one, getting divorced, or having regrets for something we've done, hard times leave us feeling broken. We conceal and hide our cracks for fear of shattering our "perfect" image. What we don't realize is that everyone has cracks. What happens with our cracks and how deep they run is determined by how and what we do to cope with them.

I want to share with you how my faith has carried me through times of brokenness, and that a broken heart can be made whole again. In every experience, there's also healing – a healing that requires patience, forgiveness, and trust in God's plan for us.

Peeling Back the Layers

As always, I compare these life-learned lessons to something in the kitchen. Let's take, for example, hard-boiling an egg. I love eating them, but the peeling process not so much. No matter how hard I try, I can never seem to get the perfect peel. Once I start, half the white layer comes off with the shell or the yolk is over or under done. As a food blogger, you can imagine how this frustrates me. How am I able to pull together a delicious meal, but demolish a hard-boiled egg? I've found that peeling the perfect hard-boiled egg begins with the cooking process and ends with practice and patience.

Similarly, we've built layers in our lives over the years; layers of fear, doubt, guilt, insecurity, resentment, and so on. These layers come from all the things in our lives that we never expected. If we peel them back with haste and impatience, we can make matters much worse for others and ourselves, but when we exercise practice and patience, we can end up with something much more beautiful.

"Of course, there is no formula for success except, perhaps, an unconditional acceptance of life and what it brings."–**Arthur Rubinstein**[3]

Rejection

One of the most exciting parts about life is that it's unpredictable. How boring would it be if we already knew the outcome of every hope and dream we ever had? For example, when I set out to write my first book, I had no idea if it would become a bestseller or if it would get lost in the mix of millions of other books. Before I would ever be able to determine the success or failure of my book, I needed to establish what my end-goal was in writing it. Was I writing it to become a bestseller or was I writing it for my own personal growth? I began to realize that the more words I put down on paper, the more I started to discover about myself.

Rejection is one example of how we can feel cracked and broken. Many people adjust their lives to filter out any kind of rejection. They want to make sure they are right in everyone else's eyes and accepted in everything they do. Trying to win the acceptance of all people is a losing battle. Everybody has different likes and dislikes; none of us are the same. One person may read this book and find it to be too short or lacking substance, while another could say they appreciated its simplicity and felt moved by what they just read. Opinions are subjective, and they encompass so many aspects of our lives—colors, fashion, politics, relationships, faith, climate— just about anything can be a platform for debate. Even more interesting is the fact that our own opinions change throughout the years. Opinions are ever-moving targets, and for this reason alone, it is impossible to obtain the acceptance of others in everything we do.

"Rejection is merely a redirection; a course correction to your destiny." – **Bryant McGill**[4]

Negative experiences, rejections, and failures do not define who we are–they redirect us. How we react to rejection is much more significant than rejection itself. These words are much easier to say than to live by.

Instead of looking at rejection as criticism and negativity, we should look for opportunities that help us grow on our path to success. While we can be rejected in our endeavors, it's even more painful when we are rejected by our peers. As I would tell my children, "If you have to change for people to like you, maybe you weren't meant to be friends." When we start questioning who we are and begin changing ourselves for the approval of others, it may be time to take a step back and decide whether it's us who needs to change or the circle of people we are engaging with. Sometimes, it can be a little bit of both.

Evaluating ourselves through the eyes of other people doesn't always have to be a negative experience. The rejection process can be an excellent breeding ground for self-awareness. Suppose we find ourselves in a conflict with another person. That person chooses to say hurtful things or no longer wants to be our friend. We could handle this situation in various ways:

1. We could walk away from that relationship with resentment and anger.
2. We could reflect on the situation and take responsibility for any hurt we may have caused the other person.
3. We could ask ourselves if it was a mutually beneficial relationship or if we are better off going our separate ways.

The first way is reactive and offers us nothing for growth. When we continue to approach things in this way, we feel less-than, not good enough, and broken; however, if we use every moment as an opportunity for reflection and growth, we will find our shells getting a bit more resilient as we grow. Exercising self-awareness doesn't mean we have to reshape who we are or conform to the standards of others; it simply means we become more mindful of our actions in future situations. Regardless of our shortcomings, there will always be people who will readily reject us, just as there will be those who will easily accept us. Seek out the latter; find *your* people. These will be the ones you can show your cracks to without feeling rejected.

"I can't tell you the key to success, but the key to failure is trying to please everyone."– **Ed Sheeran**[5]

People Pleasing

Another form of rejection can be found in people-pleasing, which often leads us to reject ourselves. We aim to please others because we yearn for their approval. We sometimes even downplay our accomplishments in things to steer away the attention.

This is not God's design for us. He wants us to take our talents and contribute to the communities we live in. Whether it be art, food, writing, singing, dancing, or something else, these are gifts from God and are meant to be celebrated and used for good. It doesn't matter who the people are that we are trying to please; pleasing others at the expense of our own happiness will never leave us feeling full.

People-pleasing starts in our childhood. As a child, we had certain needs for protection and stability. When those needs weren't met, we learned that by pleasing people that were closest to us, we were loved. People-pleasing goes a bit deeper than letting a person go ahead of us in line at the grocery store. Typically, people-pleasing comes at the expense of our own needs and self-care. We sacrifice our time and energy by putting other people's needs before our own. People-pleasing and fear of rejection go hand in hand. We want so badly to be accepted that we will do whatever we can in order to receive it. The ironic thing about this behavior is that it can actually damage relationships and set us up for unhealthy future relationships.

Perfection

For the same reasons we aim to please others and fear rejection, we strive for perfection. We do so to compensate for where we think we fall short in life. Those who seek perfection tend to be overly sensitive to the opinions of others. The truth is you can strive for perfection, but you will never fully reach it. Being perfect is a state of mind, something that differs from person to person. In everything we do, we can set goals and work hard to achieve them, but absolute perfection is unattainable, only God is perfect.

> ... *perfection is an impossible goal. Those who become preoccupied with it inevitably set themselves up for failure and psychological turmoil. They become obsessed with winning the validation of others and demonstrating their worth through flawless performance after flawless performance. They ruminate chronically about their imperfections, brood over what could have been or should have been, and experience considerable anxiety and even shame and guilt about their perceived inadequacies and unworthiness.*
>
> **- Thomas Curran and Andrew P. Hill**[6]

The article written above, "Perfectionism Is Increasing, and That's Not Good News," went on to speak about the damage that striving for perfection can cause in the lives of people young and old. Our society at large promotes perfection without us even realizing it, as we are sorted, sifted, and ranked in almost every area of life. We have milestones (crawling, walking, potty-training), grades and sports, college pursuit and acceptances, promotions, and so many other things. If we are not careful, every part of our life can turn into a competition to be perfect. We so easily call people out on their errors and their mistakes that we forget that we mess up, too!

Let me clarify. There is a difference between striving to be the best in a sport, career, hobby, or other area of our life and striving to be perfect. A good measure to distinguish between the two is by determining who we are trying to be better than. Are we in competition with others? Are we always trying to one-up someone else or be more like *that* person? Or are we reflecting on our own shortcomings and striving to continue forward to better ourselves? Striving toward perfection will produce heartache, whereas striving toward improvement will produce healthy, happier lives.

'Egg'cellent Facts & Recipes

Cracked But Not Broken could not be the title of a cookbook without eggs. Before we dive into those m'egg"nificient recipes, let's talk about all the great reasons to love them!

Did you know that eggs are not only delicious to eat but, they have also been linked to many health benefits? In 2021, VAL-CO provided "21 Fun Egg Facts for World Egg Day." Who knew there could be so many facts about eggs? You can check out the full list on their website, but here are ten of the facts I found most fascinating:

- Eggs are good for your eyes. They contain lutein, which prevents cataracts and muscle degeneration.
- Egg yolks are one of the few foods that naturally contain Vitamin D.
- Brown eggs are more expensive because the hens that lay them are larger and require more feed.
- Duck eggs are higher in fat and better for baking.
- Eggs are rich in choline, which promotes normal cell activity.
- If you drop an egg on the floor, sprinkle it heavily with salt for easy clean up.
- Eggs age more in one day at room temperature than in one week in the refrigerator.
- The fastest omelet maker in the world made 427 two-egg omelets in thirty minutes.
- The word "yolk" derives from an Old English word for "yellow." Therefore it is egg white and "egg yellow."
- There are several reasons why we commonly eat chicken eggs instead of duck or turkey eggs. Chickens lay more eggs, they need less nesting space, and they don't have the strong mothering instincts of turkeys and ducks, which makes egg collection easier.[1]

Good Egg vs Bad Egg

A quick way to determine whether or not the egg
you are about to use is good or bad:

Fill a bowl or cup with cold tap water and place your unbroken egg into
the water. An egg that sinks to the bottom and lays flat on one side is fresh
and good to eat, but an egg that floats to the top should be thrown away.

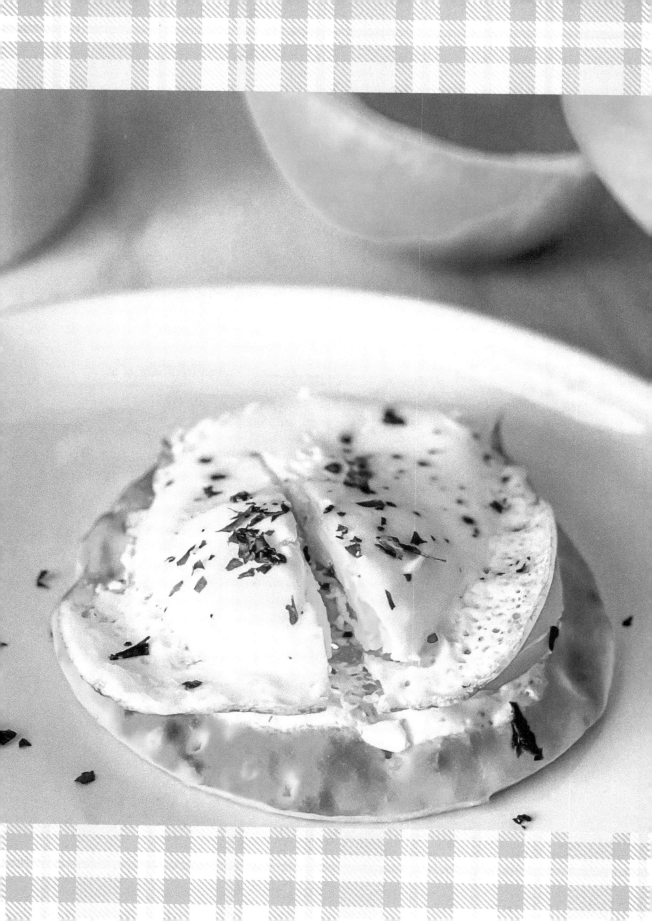

Breakfast Flatbread
With A Tangy Dill Sauce

Prep Time: 10 min. / **Cook Time:** none / **Serves:** 4

INGREDIENTS FOR FLATBREAD:

4 slices of Naan Mini Flatbread Rounds
1 tomato, thinly sliced
4 large eggs, cooked to preference
Salt and pepper, for taste

INGREDIENTS FOR LEMON DILL SAUCE:

2 Tbsps. plain Greek yogurt
1/4 tsp. garlic salt
Pinch of dried dill weed
Squeeze of lemon

INSTRUCTIONS:

1) In a small bowl, combine ingredients for lemon dill sauce.
2) Toast flatbread in a toaster oven.
3) Spread lemon dill sauce over flatbread.
4) Place a slice of tomato on each flatbread followed by cooked egg.
5) Add salt and pepper for taste.

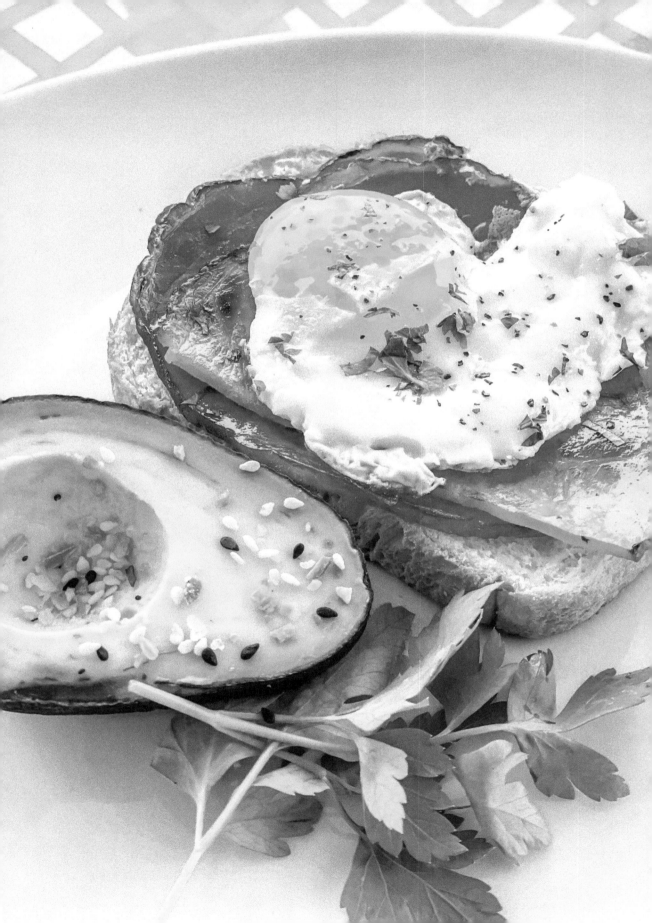

OPEN-FACED HAM AND EGG TOAST

Prep Time: 5 min. / **Cook Time:** none / **Serves:** 4

INGREDIENTS:

4 slices of thick-cut ham
4 slices of whole wheat bread
4 large eggs, cooked to preference
Fresh parsley, chopped
Salt and pepper, for taste

INSTRUCTIONS:

1) Cook ham and eggs to desired doneness.
2) Toast bread and assemble.
3) Sprinkle with fresh parsley, salt, and pepper.

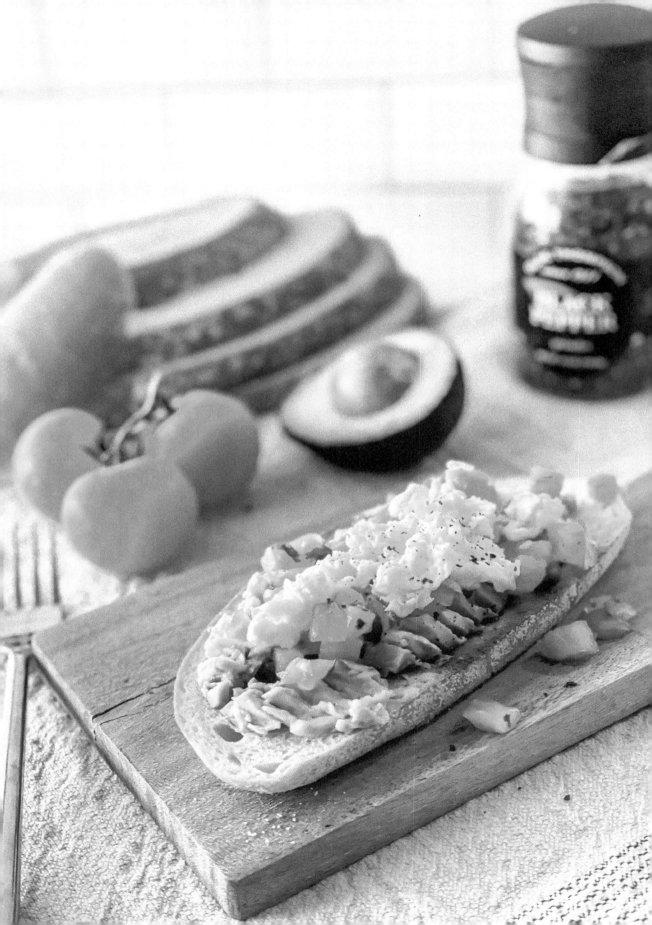

Breakfast Bruschetta

Prep Time: 10 min. / **Cook Time:** 5 min. / **Serves:** 4

Ingredients:

4 slices of French bread
1 Tbsp. unsalted butter
2 large eggs
1/8 cup milk
1/2 cup pico de gallo (diced tomatoes, onions, cilantro)
Salt and pepper, for taste
1 avocado, mashed

Instructions:

1) Preheat the oven to 400ºF.
2) Melt butter and brush it on both sides of French bread. Arrange on a baking sheet and bake each side for 3-5 minutes until toasted. Remove from the oven and set it aside.
3) In a medium bowl, whisk together the eggs, milk, salt and pepper.
4) Place a nonstick skillet over medium-low heat. Add cooking spray to the pan and pour in the eggs. Stir until eggs are scrambled to your desired consistency.
5) Spread a portion of the mashed avocado on one side of each slice of toasted bread. Top with scrambled egg and pico de gallo.

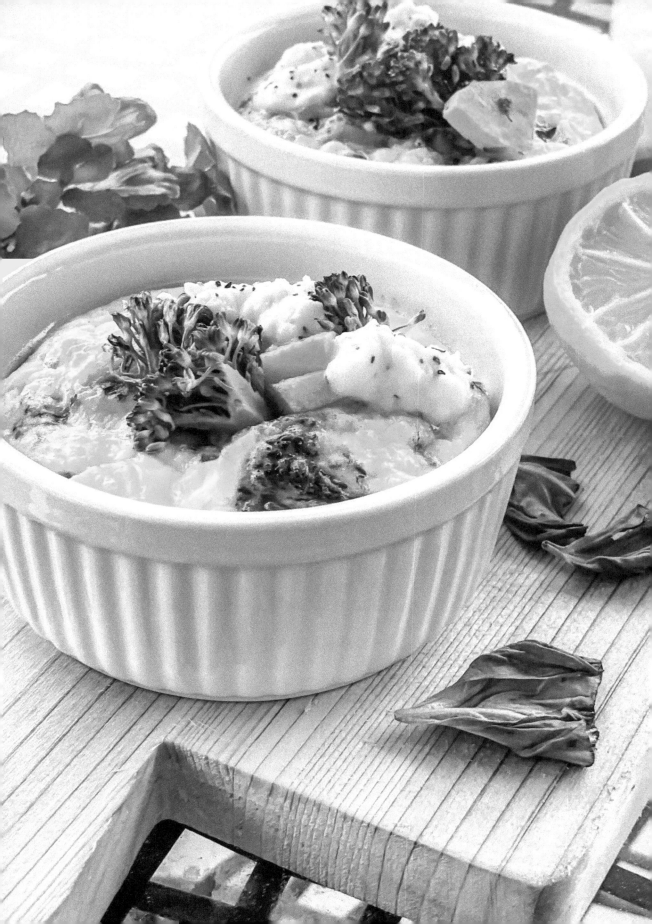

Sweet Potato Frittata

Prep Time: 20 min. / **Cook Time:** 30 min. / **Serves:** 2-4

Ingredients:

1 large sweet potato
1 cup finely chopped broccoli
1/4 cup ricotta cheese, plus 1 extra Tbsp.
4 large eggs
1/2 lemon, juiced
1/2 Tbsp. basil, finely chopped
2 Tbsps. extra-virgin olive oil
Salt and pepper, for taste

Instructions:

1) Preheat the oven to 350ºF.
2) Lightly spray two porcelain ramekins or small oven-safe dishes, and place on a baking sheet.
3) Peel and dice the sweet potato into bite-sized pieces (approximately 1/2 inch cubes).
4) In a medium skillet, heat olive oil.
5) Add sweet potatoes, salt, and pepper, and stir to coat all pieces. Add chopped broccoli, mix well. Cook for 15-20 minutes, stirring occasionally to prevent burning. Cook until soft enough to pierce with a fork. Remove from heat and divide the sweet potato mixture between two ramekins or small oven safe dish.
6) In a medium bowl, whisk eggs along with ricotta cheese and fresh basil. Pour egg mixture over vegetables in two ramekins or small dishes. Bake in the oven for 25-30 minutes. Meanwhile, combine lemon juice with remaining ricotta cheese, salt, and pepper.
7) Top each ramekin or small dish with lemon ricotta and serve.

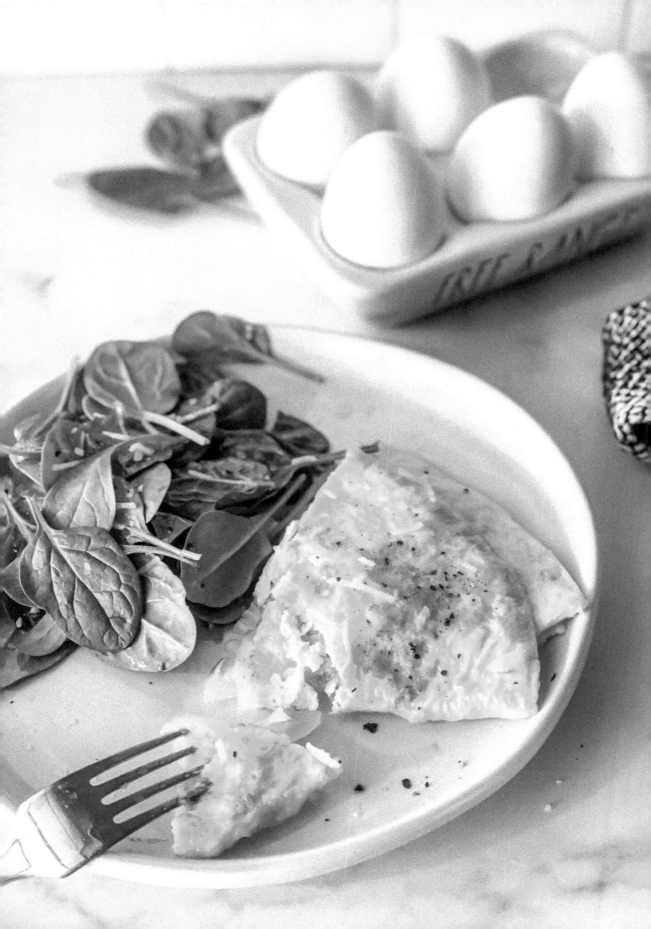

Classic Omelet and Greens

Prep Time: 5 min. / **Cook Time:** 5 min. / **Serves:** 1-2

Ingredients:

2 Tbsps. olive oil, divided
1/4 cup yellow onion, finely chopped
2-3 large eggs
1 tsp. water
Sea salt and cracked black pepper
1/4 cup Parmesan cheese, finely grated
2 Tbsps. fresh lemon juice
3 oz. baby spinach

Instructions:

1) Heat 1 tablespoon of oil in large nonstick skillet on medium heat. Add onion and sauté until soft and translucent, then set aside.
2) In a medium bowl, whisk eggs together. Add water, and pour into heated skillet with onions.
3) Allow eggs to set and reduce heat to low. Cover until cooked through. Sprinkle salt, pepper, and Parmesan cheese over top. Fold in half.
4) In a medium bowl, combine the remaining oil with lemon juice, cracked pepper, and sea salt. Toss spinach greens to coat. Sprinkle with Parmesan cheese and serve with omelet.

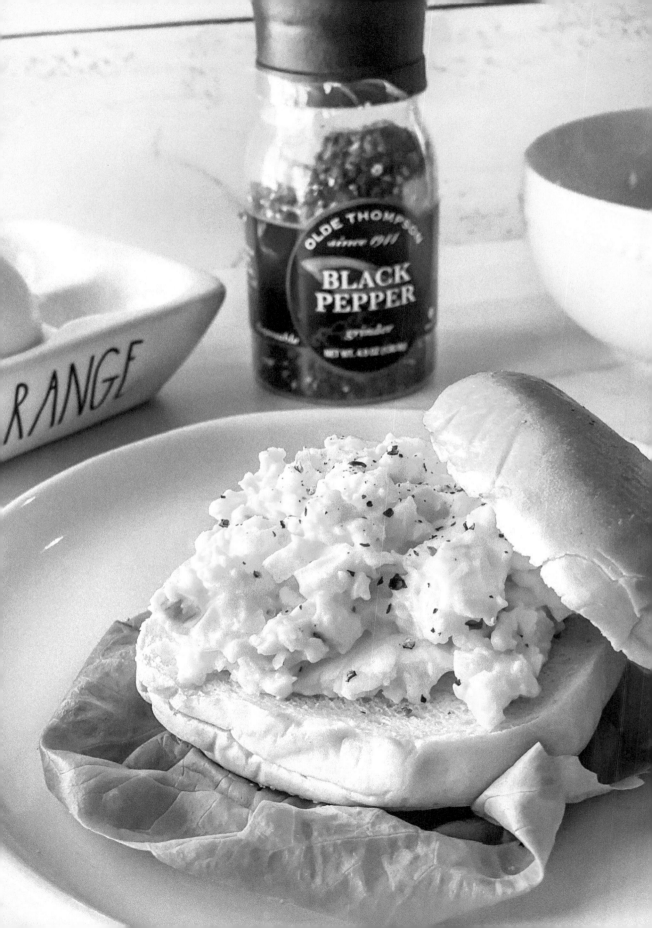

Egg Salad Bagel Sandwich

Prep Time: 10 min. / **Cook Time:** none / **Serves:** 1-2

Ingredients:

3 hard-boiled eggs, chopped
2 Tbsps. low-fat mayonnaise
1 celery stalk, diced
1 green onion, sliced
Salt and pepper, for taste
Bagel, lightly toasted

Instructions:

1) In a medium bowl, combine eggs, mayonnaise, green onion, and celery. Add salt and pepper for taste.
2) Serve on a lightly toasted bagel and enjoy!

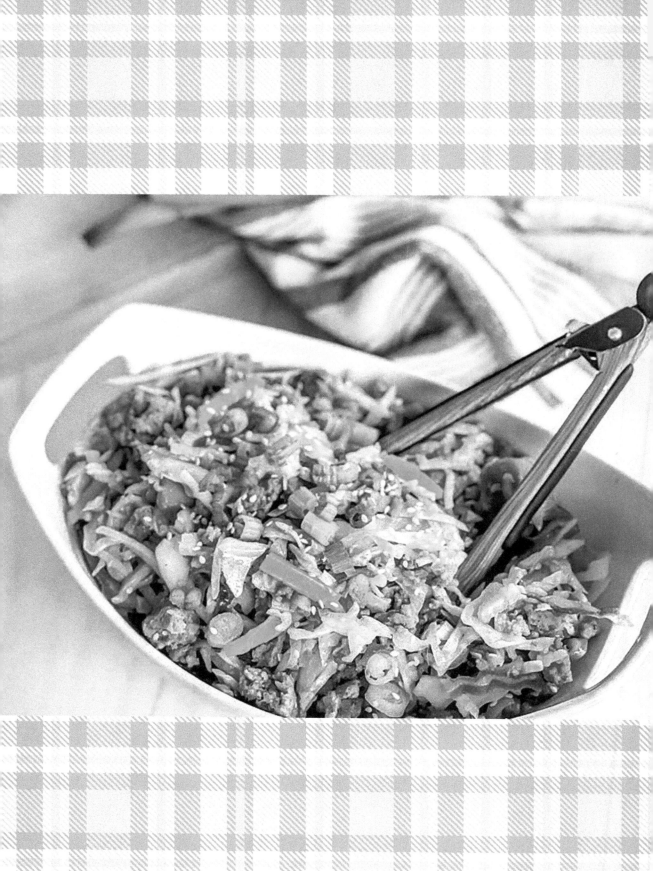

Egg Roll in a Bowl

Prep Time: 5 min. / **Cook Time:** 20 min. / **Serves:** 2-3

Ingredients:

1 lb. ground sweet Italian sausage
1 bag (16 oz.) of coleslaw mix
1 tsp. avocado or sesame oil
3 Tbsps. liquid coconut aminos (soy sauce substitute)
1/2 tsp. Sriracha
1 Tbsp. rice vinegar
1/3 cup yellow onion, diced
2 Tbsps. garlic, minced
2 large green onions, sliced
1/2 tsp. ginger paste
Salt and pepper, for taste
Sesame seeds

Instructions:

1) In a large skillet over medium heat, add oil, garlic, and yellow onion. Cook until soft and translucent.
2) Add sausage, salt, pepper, ginger paste, and Sriracha. Cook until meat is crumbled and no longer pink.
3) Add coleslaw mix, liquid aminos, and rice vinegar. Cook until coleslaw is soft.
4) Top with green onions and sesame seeds.

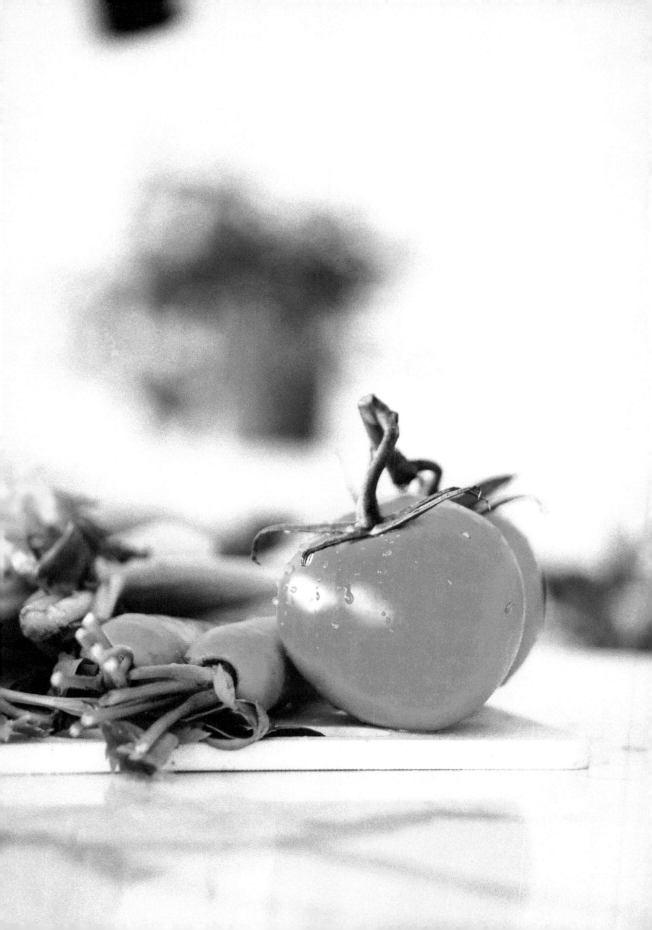

Pressure Cooked

"No pressure is greater than God's power."
– Charles R. Swindoll [8]

PRESSURE COMES FROM VARIOUS THINGS WE FACE. FROM school to our relationships to our jobs and more, pressure surrounds every aspect of what we do. Handling and managing pressure is critical for our mental health. Stress is the product of pressure and can leave us cracked.

Not only do everyday pressures agonize us, but there are so many unforeseen variables. For example, you may have spent years dedicated to your job when suddenly you're faced with a company lay-off. Or you've strived to lead a balanced healthy lifestyle and you receive a devastating diagnosis.

Pressure can either work for us or against us. Sometimes it can consume our thoughts and lead us into depression and anxiety. Other times, it can clarify our priorities and make us realize what needs our time and attention. Pressure can also create psychological harm through mental and emotional distress when it is ignored. It is important to recognize and understand where your pressures come from and whether they can be managed better.

Parent Guilt

There is no pressure on earth like that of being a parent. Many parents experience moments where they feel as if they are failing their children. From the first time I became a mom, I felt pressures that I needed to do everything right. From providing structured activities to bedtime routines, the pressures of parenting and decision-making have been endless.

Eventually, I learned there wasn't a right or wrong way to parent in every situation. Though the pressure to do right by our children stems from love, it is not in line with God's desire for us as parents. Allowing this kind of pressure to persist in our parenting robs us from joy, contentment, and all of the other beautiful parts of parenthood.

Guilt is a form of rejecting ourselves. When we compare ourselves to another, there will always be something we can do differently or possibly better. It doesn't take away from the fact that we love our children. More importantly as parents, we need to decide who we are striving to please. If our end goal is to raise happy, healthy, and kind human beings, then perhaps we don't need anyone else's approval but our own.

"The very fact that you worry about being a good mom means that you already are one." - **Jodi Picoult**[9]

For single and working parents who feel they can't do enough, the guilt can be unbearable. If this applies to you, know that your child is loved by you and that is all that matters. Just because you can't attend career day or a field trip to the museum does not take away from the loving, caring amazing mom (or dad) that you are.

Breast-feeding or bottle-feeding, co-sleeping or crib sleeping, screen time or no screen time, snacks before or after dinner, dating at thirteen or sixteen.. these are just some of the many choices we must make as a parent. No matter what choice we make, there will always someone there to tell us why their decision is better. Oh, the shame of guilt. It's awful! And the worst part is that nobody has the right answer for your child except *you*. You are the one who knows them better than anyone else. Yes, there is a huge chance you might not get it right, quite a few times, but that shouldn't be the focus. Make the most of every moment you can with your child, but don't beat yourself up over the small stuff.

Worry

Another thing that can overwhelm us, but is not limited to parents, is worry. There are many things that can cause us to worry: uncertainty in the workplace, traumatic events, sickness, and many others. Almost anything which could cause us to worry could be summed up in this one attribute: it's out of our control. Failure is probably one of the biggest worries most of us struggle with. We need to give ourselves room to breathe and room to fail. Failure is not the end of the world.

To worry about things we can't change is a terrible waste of emotional energy. Rather than worry, people who go the distance have learned the art of "creative anxiety." While worry is destructive, creative anxiety is constructive. Worry focuses on the problem; creative anxiety focuses on the solution. Worry controls us; creative anxiety puts us in control of our emotions. – **Ed Rowell, "Learn to Drop the Worry Habit"** [10]

As I mentioned, anything can have a negative tone with rejection and guilt, but these things can also have positive effects on our lives if we allow them to. Worry often transforms into stress, anxiety, depression, and many other negative things for our health and well-being. It can also lead to many complications in our physical and mental health. Rather than ignoring concerns which cause us worry, we should learn to talk through them with trusted individuals.

Cracks, no matter what they have been caused by, are more likely to spread and become much harder to repair the longer we wait to address them.

"Instead of worrying about what you cannot control, shift your energy to what you can create."–**Roy T. Bennett** [11]

PRESSURE COOKING TIPS AND DISHES

Talk about pressure.. who doesn't love the convenience of cooking with a pressure cooker? Snacks, breakfast, lunch, dinner—it seems almost anything can be thrown into the pot for a quick and easy meal solution. Here are some helpful tips and tricks to get the most from your pressure cooker (Please note that some of these tips directly refer to the Instant Pot® brand):

1. Use at least half a cup of liquid when pressure cooking.

A pressure cooker uses steam to build pressure that ultimately cooks the food. To create that pressure, the inner pot <u>must have at least half to one cup of liquid</u>. This is the only way to pressurize the unit, and it's a crucial tip you'll want to remember.

2. Use liquids other than water to add flavor.

Adding flavorful liquids like broths, juices, and stocks can add a ton of flavor to your dishes. You can turn basic rice into a flavorful side simply by swapping the water with a mix of tomato broth and chicken broth and then adding in a bit of sauteed onions and garlic. Or, you can add flavor to your chicken by swapping the water for chicken broth.[12]

3. If your pressure cooker overflows…

When filling your pot with food and liquid, you should keep in mind that your ingredients will expand and can cause the venting knob to clog, leading to liquid spilling over.

Pay close attention to the "max" line and make sure to remain below it.[13]

4. How to clean the silicone ring.

If you find that the ring is holding onto food odors–even after you've washed it–fill the pressure cooker with two cups of vinegar or water and lemon rind. Then run it on the "steam" setting for two minutes. Good as new![14]

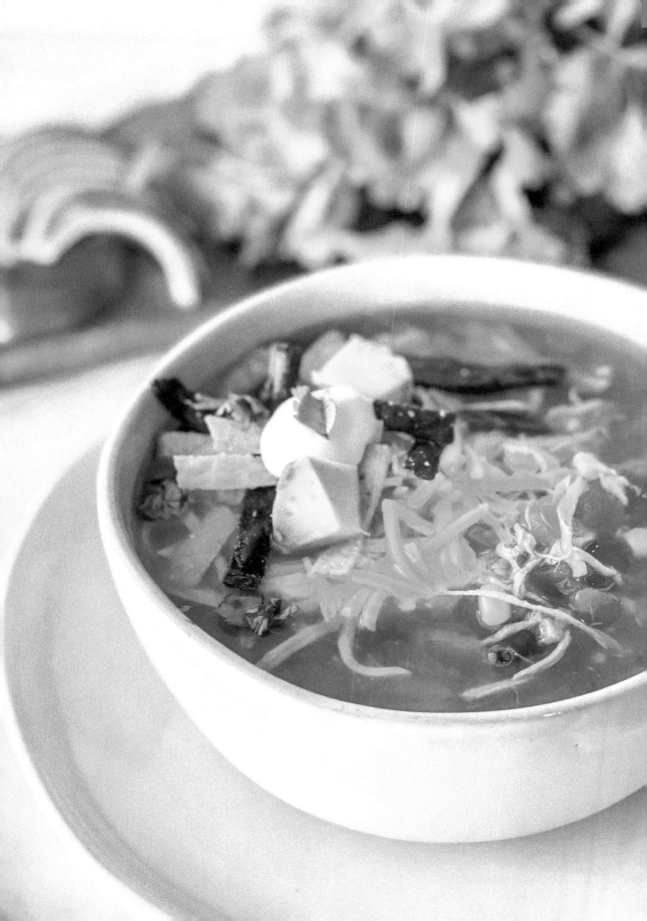

PRESSURE COOKED CHICKEN TORTILLA SOUP

Prep Time: 5 min. / **Cook Time:** 25 min. / **Serves:** 4

INGREDIENTS:

1 (32 oz.) container low-sodium chicken broth
2 (10 oz.) cans diced tomatoes with green chiles
1 lb. skinless, boneless chicken breast
1 (15 oz.) can black beans, drained
1 (10 oz.) can green enchilada sauce
1 (10 oz.) package frozen corn
1/2 red onion, diced
2 Tbsp. garlic, minced
1 tsp. ground cumin
1 tsp. salt
1/4 tsp. black pepper
Chili powder, for taste
*Garnish of choice

INSTRUCTIONS:

1) Place all ingredients in a pressure cooker.
2) Close and lock the lid. Be sure the pressure valve is closed.
3) Select a setting according to the manufacturer's instructions. Set the timer for 15 minutes.
4) After set cooking time, release the pressure according to the manufacturer's instructions for about 10 minutes. Unlock and remove the lid.
5) Carefully remove chicken from the pot (it will be hot!). Shred and place back into the pot.
6) Stir and serve with garnish of choice.

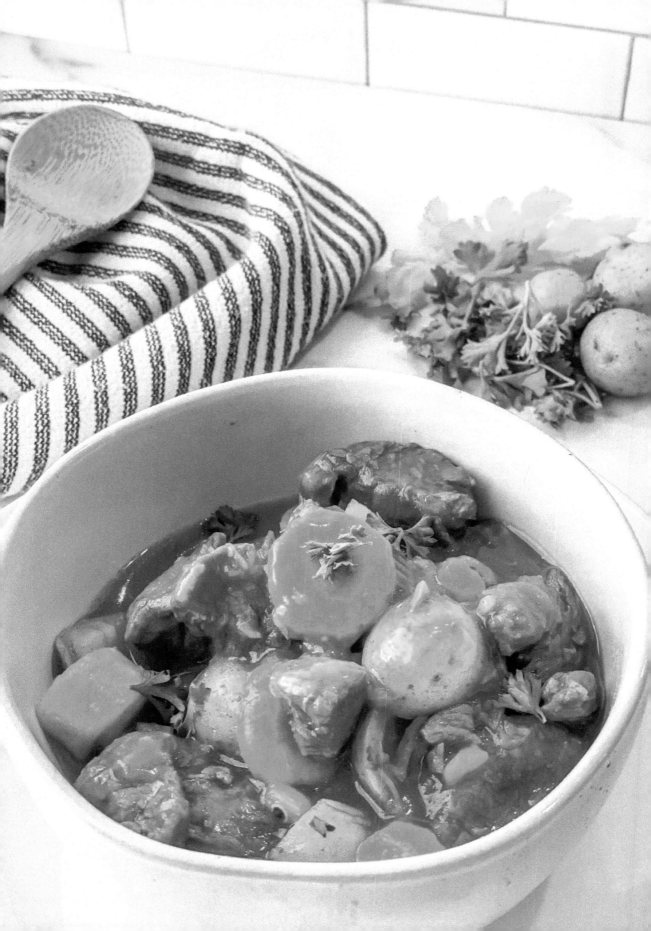

Pressure Cooked Beef Stew

Prep Time: 10 min. / **Cook Time:** 35 min. / **Serves:** 4

Ingredients:

2 cups low-sodium beef stock
1 Tbsp. olive oil
1 yellow onion, sliced
1 Tbsp. garlic, minced
4 carrots, diced into rounds
3 cups small golden potatoes, halved
2 lbs. cubed beef stew meat
2 ribs of celery, sliced into pieces
1 Tbsp. Worcestershire sauce
2 tsps. cornstarch
2 Tbsps. cold water
1 packet onion soup mix
Salt and pepper, for taste
2 tsps. fresh parsley

Instructions:

1) Turn on pressure cooker and select the sauté function according to the manufacturer's instructions. Place olive oil and beef cubes inside inner pot and brown all sides for about 5 minutes (stirring frequently).
2) Add diced vegetables, beef stock, onion soup mix, garlic, and 1 teaspoon of fresh parsley. Stir to combine.
3) Close and lock lid. Select soup/stew function. Set cooking time to 35 minutes and allow to pressurize (be sure steam valve is closed).
4) In a small bowl, combine cornstarch, Worcestershire sauce, and water. Set aside.
5) Release pressure and remove lid. Stir in cornstarch mixture to thicken sauce.
6) Add salt and pepper for taste and serve with remaining parsley.

The Deepest Cracks

"Father, I don't understand what you are doing but I know your plan is greater."
- Wendy Blight[15]

WHILE THERE ARE SOME EXPERIENCES IN LIFE WHICH leave small cracks, we cannot overlook the experiences that can leave much deeper, long-lasting cracks, such as trauma and grief. These two topics often affect us at such an intimate level we are unable to express or process exactly how we feel. They often take much more time to work through, but these are some of the most important cracks we address.

Trauma

We can all relate to experiencing some form of trauma in our lives. To be honest, the COVID pandemic has been a collective trauma crisis in the making. If nothing else, it has surely played a role in traumatizing our mental health. The impact of worry and anxiety over COVID-19 has been overwhelming. The up and down roller coaster of emotions can't even begin to describe how difficult the past two years have been for a good portion of the world.

COVID-19 has interrupted our daily routines, created high levels of uncertainty, and taken the lives of many people we love. It is no surprise we have been left feeling sad, angry, and frustrated. Trauma is described as a psychological result of an exposure, incident, or event that has lasting adverse effects on our mental, physical, social, emotional, and/or spiritual well-being. Simply put, it's not easy.

"Trauma creates change you didn't choose; healing is about creating change you do choose." **– Michelle Rosenthall**[16]

Picture that hard-boiled egg we talked about in the first chapter. If there had been any sort of crack in the shell during the boiling process, the yolk would have boiled itself out of the egg. This would result in the egg no longer looking the same as it did before it went into the pot. Trauma affects the mind in a similar way. When a person experiences trauma, they no longer look the same as they once did. It is possible, depending on the type and severity of trauma, that their physical appearance would seem the same as it was before, but how they process things moving forward would be drastically different. Trauma comes with various levels of damage that can leave us with permanent cracks.

My faith tells me that God can still bring something good from a difficult situation. Jennifer Bricker is an American acrobat who was born without any legs. Nick Vujicic was born without legs or arms. Both of them go all over the world, spreading their messages of hope. There are many more people who have been born with disabilities, faced unforeseen accidents, or found themselves plagued by illness but have stood up and continued on with life. This is not an easy thing to do, but knowing God is working all things for the good of those who love Him is certainly some firm comfort to hold onto.

Some of us are exposed to trauma due to the evil intentions of others like abuse, neglect, greed or even natural disasters which rip away the life we once knew. No matter how trauma may come our way, there are thousands upon thousands of stories of people who have survived what they would consider their darkest moments. Instead of succumbing to the trauma, we can use the testimony of other's experiences to overcome our own difficult times. Joining support groups, reading books, and surrounding ourselves with people who know and understand the type of trauma we are going through can help us navigate through our own difficult time and offer us words of wisdom.

Grief

Unfortunately, I learned what grief was at a young age. Losing a parent has been one of the deepest cracks of my life. Death is a crack that can lead us to a place of brokenness if we don't find ways to grieve in a way that promotes healing. We can do this by seeking counseling, joining support groups, or participating in charitable events that our loved one was passionate about. Surrounding ourselves with friends and family helps bring back a sense of their presence. We can honor their life by sharing all of the wonderful traits that made them so special to us.

In the last two years, I have watched my children experience similar cracks. Both have lost close friends much too soon in their short lives. As a parent, I do what I can to ensure my children don't have to experience these kinds of deep cracks, though in the case of death, it's much out of my control. Losing someone we love to death is the deepest crack of the human experience. It creates a much deeper level of pain than we even know how to comprehend.

"Death leaves a heartache no one can heal, love leaves a memory no one can steal."
- Richard Puz[17]

There are five stages that typically accompany grief: denial, anger, bargaining, depression, and acceptance. While this may be true, grief still looks and feels different for everyone. Each of us experience grief in our own way, through support groups, self-help books, or counseling services. Although these methods can help ease the heaviness of our grief, there is no set timeline of how long grief will last. When I experienced grief, I leaned on my faith. I still do, to this very day. Although it has been over thirty years since my father's passing, grief never fully goes away.

In her book, *Lost to Darkness; Enlightened by Grace*, Laura Gabriella spoke about a grief I would think to be unimaginable: the loss of her twelve-year-old son, Zachary, to suicide. She went through a roller coaster of emotions, never imagining this would one day be her life. Laura used the grief she was experiencing to fuel a non-profit focused on preventing other families from experiencing this kind of pain. Marshmallow's Hope focuses on offering counseling services and instilling the hope to continue on another day in everyone they come in contact with. While Laura advocates strongly for counseling and proper mental health care, she also speaks very passionately about the faith that has allowed her to carry on:

> *However, if you're willing to seek help outside of this world, there is a God who can transform your sorrow into an unspeakable joy. He can turn your unrest into a peace that is unspeakably indescribable. Accepting Jesus Christ as your savior, will 100 percent transform your life, take away your pain, and guide you to your purpose.*
>
> *I'm not trying to sell you something. I say this out of my own personal experience. No matter how much of a screw up I think I am, He is always right by my side despite my imperfections. I handed the wheel over to Him when I thought I couldn't drive anymore and I'm so glad I did. He has taken me down roads I never knew existed. He has given me a peace and joy that I never would have thought I could experience again.* **(Laura Gabriella, *Lost to Darkness; Enlightened by Grace*, 183-184)**

Losing someone, no matter the circumstances surrounding their death, can be a traumatic experience. We all know death is a part of life, but when it happens to someone we love, we have a hard time grasping how we move on. For many of us, we are left feeling heartbroken and we don't know how we will ever move beyond the loss.

"A broken heart heals when we allow the healing to go as deep as the wound went."–**Beth Moore**[19]

In the aftermath of death and trauma, it is okay to feel angry, frustrated, sad, and scared. Overcoming these feelings can take some diligent hard work, but that does not mean we cannot get to a place where we feel a little more whole again. Use the resources you have available to you, including some of the recommendations listed at the end of this book. Remind yourself that in these wounded moments, we find our true strength. The cracks of our trauma will not break us because believe it or not, our shells are strengthening in our weakest moments.

"Perhaps they are not stars but rather openings in heaven where the love of our lost ones pours through and shines down upon us to let us know they are happy."–**Eskimo Proverb**[18]

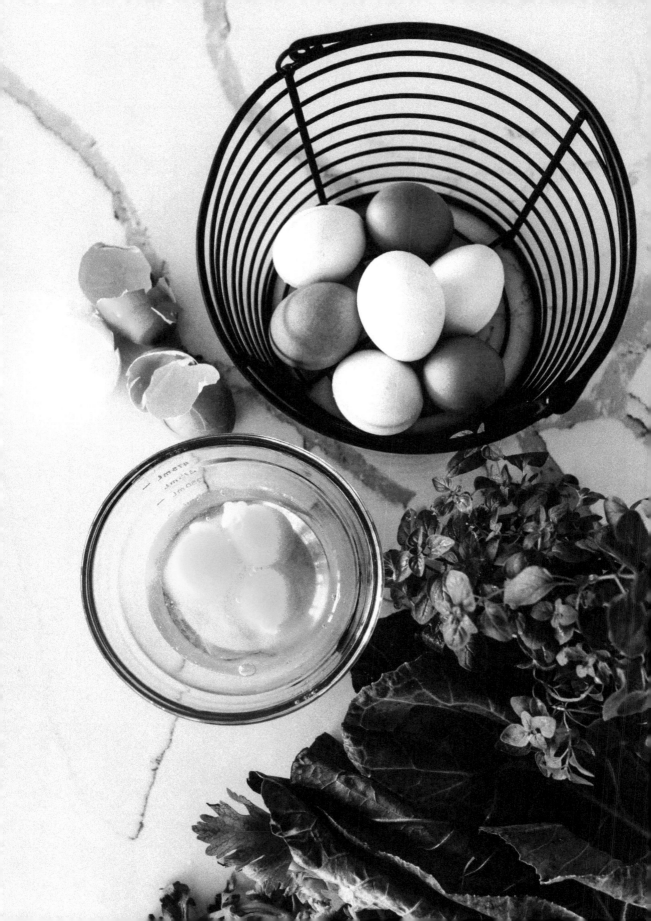

4

All Yolks Aside:
Sifting Through Relationships

*"If you want to change the way people respond to you,
change the way you respond to people."*
–Timothy Leary[20]

RELATIONSHIPS OF ANY KIND ARE NOT EASY TO NAVIGATE and can leave cracks of betrayal and heartache. The most complicated thing about relationships is people. Each of us have our own personalities, our own cracks, and our own ways of approaching life in general. All of this can make it hard to navigate with each other. If we are someone who struggles with fears of abandonment or jealousy, we could dream up complications for our relationships which don't exist. On that same note, if we are confident in who we are, we could assume that everyone feels this way and miss offering words of encouragement to those who struggle with insecurity. There are many ways in which people are different, but there is one way we are all the same: we long to be loved, accepted, and appreciated.

*"Our worst fault is our preoccupation with the faults of others."***–Khali Gibran**[21]

In the previous chapters, we talked about how we are not perfect people. We each carry cracks of our own, and we recognize that mistakes are going to happen. We wish to be shown grace in these situations, but we are not always willing to return the favor. The impatient driver riding our bumper, the annoyed cashier who had a long day... We find ourselves frustrated with people who do things just like we do sometimes.

I would be lying if I said I have never gotten too close to the car in front of me or that I have never had a bad day at work. Trying to look beyond our first reaction to these circumstances can remind us to be more forgiving and allow some grace.

"Forgiveness is an option that's more powerful than any amount of worldly shame – an option that sets us free." – **Christine Caine**[22]

The human race is quick to criticize and shame, but very slow to forgive. The Bible tells us that we are all sinners. Yes, even Christ followers make bad decisions. By extending grace and having an open mind, we just might find ourselves making deeper, more meaningful connections with other people. I, myself, have faced hard situations with other people. Feelings of resentment, anger, jealousy are all things that can crack our shell and lead us to a place of brokenness. I look to God in these moments to remind myself that I can do better.

"God promises to bring good from the storms of devastation in our lives." –**Debbie McDaniel**[23]

Broken relationships are often the outcome of misunderstandings and differing perspectives. All too often we fail to recognize that we all see and feel things differently. Being accountable for the role we play in relational hardships can build and strengthen our character. If and when we crack in a relationship, we need to learn from it, grow from it, and build from it to be a better human being.

Me, Myself, and I

The main focus, along with the problems we have in some of our relationships is the "me" mentality. When we focus solely on ourselves, we often miss the needs of others. The "me" mentality is our default mode of survival. We enter the world crying for our needs to be met. If we are not careful, we can find ourselves stuck in this immature way of thinking. Instead of considering what we can contribute, we continue focusing on what we can gain. This kind of mindset will quickly have us labeled as selfish or self-centered in our relationships.

"The most important relationship you will ever have is the one with yourself." - **Diane Von Furstenberg**[24]

Alternatively, we need to make sure we look out for ourselves so we can build long-lasting healthy relationships. What's the difference?

Have you ever sat through flight safety instructions on an airplane? Whenever they get to the part where you need to put your mask on before helping others in an emergency, I immediately think about my children. I don't think I could put myself before them if that ever were to happen. Thankfully, I've never been put to the test, but it gets me thinking about how easy it can be to put other people's needs before our own.

Contrary to what most people might think, the "me" mentality isn't all a bad thing. As I mentioned earlier, it is meant to mature. We must understand when it is time to take a break and recharge. If we overwork ourselves, we are less likely to be able to assist with the needs of others.

Labeling

So much of how we view ourselves comes from the way others make us feel. And the way we feel and view ourselves changes the way we interact with people. It becomes a vicious cycle.

> *"We must reject not only the stereotypes that others have of us but also those that we have of ourselves."*–**Shirley Chisholm**[25]

For example, one way we divide ourselves and create friction in relationships is through labeling. Making assumptions about people based on their views or the view of others. Political, religious, or gender debates are just examples of many things that crack and divide us. Like perfection, labeling is subjective to our own personal biases. We can find ourselves in relationships with two very different views, which have the potential of escalating to a point that cannot be resolved.

> *"Be the woman who fixes another woman's crown without telling the world that it was crooked."* – **Cici B.**[26]

Labels come at us in all shapes and sizes and can sometimes be the result of a situation that escalates beyond the individual(s) involved. For example, when something bad happens between two people, but one of them chooses to share their version of the story with others, they suddenly place a label on that individual to people who they've never even met. We see this happening in our world all around us. The media constantly tells us how to feel about other people by broadcasting their failures and passing judgement on strangers. You can't pull up the internet without reading an article that criticizes someone for something they did.

Labels–they absolutely crack and divide us as people.

Oftentimes, labels or assumptions come from a place of insecurity. When we label others, we do it to convince ourselves and everyone else that we are "not that." We see it in our kids' schools through cliques and exclusive friendships; we see it in our adulthood at work and in social circles. One person decides to label another by their behaviors or characteristics and suddenly, others make the same assumption without truly knowing if it's even true. What's worse is that it's difficult to navigate away from a label once it's been given.

Sometimes we even label ourselves. When you believe that you can't change something in your life because you're not "good enough" or "smart enough," you limit yourself from your true potential. Labeling does no one any good. Challenge yourself to look beyond the label, whether it be your own or someone else's.

Children

Another complication in relationships is the one which spans across generations. The millennial cannot quite understand why Grandma is always reminiscing about the "good ol' days." How could things be great back before streaming movies and handheld computers? Was it really *fun* playing with rocks in the dirt? It's hard to find commonality between people who have lived such different lives from each other.

My husband was raised as a farmer. His days started and ended with milking cows, mucking the stalls, and working the fields. His perspective on life is very different from mine. At times, this created waves in our marriage with how we parented. While I agree that hard work is an acquired trait, I sometimes feel it isn't fair for us to expect our kids to grow up the exact same way we did. It reminds me of the classic old saying, "Back when I was a kid, I had to walk to school uphill both ways barefoot in the snow." Did anyone actually ever do this?

Adults come across and interact with children in all settings—restaurants, grocery stores, schools, parks, everywhere. Whenever we take the time to speak with younger generations, we should be careful not to downplay how they feel. Many of us block out the difficulties we faced as children and only seem to remember the good times. For this reason, we sometimes forget how devastating life can be when our favorite toy breaks, our crush asks out someone else, or our best friend moves to a new school. Children are nothing more than smaller versions of ourselves. They want love, acceptance, and validation.

> *"Encourage and support your kids because children are apt to live up to what you believe of them."* –**Lady Bird Johnson**[27]

As adults, it's our responsibility to educate and inform our kids without expecting them to conform. If our children pick up a belief system, no matter the subject—faith, politics, education, equality—based on what they are told to do, rather than being allowed to ask questions and choose for themselves, eventually their belief system will crumble. Instead, children should be well-informed and properly guided to make their own decisions.

Children also need to see that relationships are imperfect. There will be differences of opinion, and not everyone will think and feel the same way we do. Teaching our children this life lesson can greatly benefit them throughout their lives in school, in friendships, and even in marriage one day.

Children need adults—parents, grandparents, teachers, friends, mentors—in their lives who are willing to allow them room to learn and grow; adults who will be delicate with the cracks they are facing and will help guide them to a sense of wholeness.

Marriage

What relationship could be more complicated than the one we share with our spouse? Our spouses see the very best and the very worst of us... maybe all within the same day. Whether you're newly married or have been together for years, each marriage has its ups and downs. Being happily married doesn't look like a storybook, although at times we expect it to. A good marriage consists of two people who are committed to loving and supporting one another. Like any relationship, marriage takes hard work, healthy communication, realistic expectations, and respect for each other. These are the foundational building blocks to a happy and fulfilled marriage.

"In life, it's not where you go, it's who you travel with." **–Charles Schulz**[28]

Contrary to the ball-and-chain theory, marriage is not all bad. It is the beginning of new adventures. My husband is my person; he's my other half. Although we've had some bumps in our road, we're blessed to be on this journey together. With each milestone, we learn more about ourselves and each other. We're willing to grow through what we go through, and in doing so, we have established a deeper, more intimate kind of love. I believe that those who seek perfection in their marriage will never find it.

"You don't love someone because they're perfect, you love them in spite of the fact that they're not." **–Jodi Picoult**[29]

Marriage is about accepting our differences and remembering that God uniquely designed us just the way we are. Showing all of ourselves to the other person, the good, the bad, the cracks, and still knowing that we are deeply loved and accepted by that person.

This is not to say that all circumstances in marriage are easy. Infidelity, addiction, and abuse are things that can cause damage to a marriage, which can feel irreparable or broken. Couples therapy and relationship counseling can help mitigate some of these difficulties. If you feel that your marriage is damaged beyond repair, it is important to note that choosing divorce is a major life decision that should never be taken lightly. Seeking professional help can provide guidance for how to navigate through such a difficult time.

Family

My husband and I have a blended family with children from previous marriages as well as one together. This has been challenging at times because what we believed was right for discipline, encouragement, and growth was not always in sync. Now that our kids have grown, we've learned how to compromise on our differences and make adjustments when necessary. Blending a family takes time and patience, but with commitment and acceptance, it can be a really beautiful part of life.

"Families are like fudge, mostly sweet with lots of nuts." –**Les Dawson**[30]

Whether you have a conventional family or one that is completely unorthodox, your family makes you *you*. Just as all of the previous sections have mentioned, relationships of all kinds are complicated. The relationships most of us seem to struggle with more than any other is with those closest to us: our parents, siblings, spouses, children, and relatives.

Think about your family. Perhaps you have a family member you don't fully understand or feel connected with. This division may come through conflicting beliefs, divided tastes, varied hobbies, or even age gaps. You might not understand why someone would spend money on hiking equipment, and they might not understand why you would spend money on hand-painted serving dishes. We *all* have our differences. I encourage you not to allow family differences to become cracks that span and divide. Instead, focus on finding common ground, and learn how to love each other well.

"Family is not an important thing, it's everything." –**Michael J. Fox**[31]

Building Relationships Around The Table

Building a relationship takes effort but it doesn't have to be complicated. A meal gathered around the table can be one way of strengthening that bond. For many families today, dinner time is a brief moment between events. Work schedules and sports schedules often collide, making a traditional meal next to impossible. There are many benefits which come from a family sitting down to have dinner together that should not be overlooked.

Family meals can benefit both parents and children in the following ways:

- Allows parents to connect on a deeper level with their children by engaging in conversation
- Creates a supportive environment that encourages togetherness
- Children are more likely to eat healthy, well-balanced meals
- Promotes bonding within sibling relationships
- Strengthens relationships overall[32]

Most families know and understand these benefits, but still find themselves with the dilemma of limited time at their dinner tables. Here are some ideas which might help create some solutions:

Meal Prep

Having healthy meals ready to go can save time for families on the go. Meal prepping can also help save money at the grocery store. In some instances, this will eliminate the prep time and allow the family to enjoy a meal together. In all instances, this will ensure the family is receiving more nutrition than they would find at a drive-thru window.

Create Special Memories

What happens when one child needs to go to basketball practice and another has a band recital at the same time? Get creative with your family meals. If there are only one or two nights a week when everyone in the family can sit down together, protect those nights and make it happen. If you must take a child to practice and your spouse stays home with the other children, make the most of those moments, as well. Sometimes, families focus on the family unit only as a whole. Remember, each person is a vital part of the family. Parents should rotate their time with the children to help build that trust as a role model in the child's life. A Norman Rockwell picture perfect moment is not required to create special memories; all that is needed is a parent sitting down and conversing with their child. Special memories can be created anywhere as long as there is a will to do so.

Prioritizing

If there are too many events to find even one evening of family time together, it may signify a need to check the calendar for priorities. This is not meant to condemn, but to be used as a reflection. As parents, we all too often focus on all the extra activities our children can be enrolled in to give them an advantage for their future. Never forget, the most important advantage for your child's future is a solid relationship with you, their parent. When all the sports are over and dance lessons have ended, they will need someone to turn to for advice. An excellent way to ensure you are established as this resource is to make sure you have quality talks and time spent with your child. These can be held anywhere, but the dinner table always seems to be a neutral environment. People tend to relax a little more when they are eating good food.

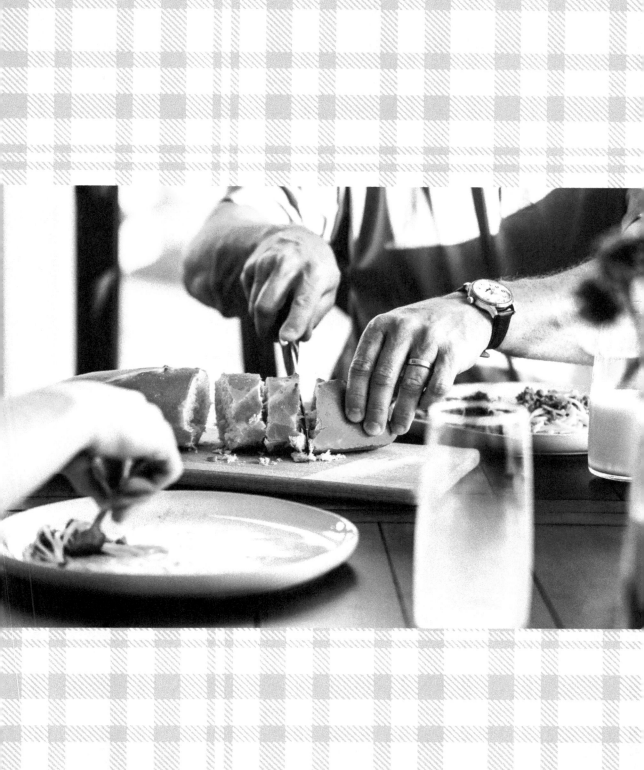

Game Nights, Crafts & Traditions

Your children won't remember all of the things you said or did in their life, but they will remember the memories you created *together*. Game night, craft sessions, and family traditions can lead to a family bonding experience that is not only fun, but can improve your child's mental and emotional development. Friday night pizza with cards or Sunday afternoon crafting are fun ways to carve out special time with your kids. Board games such as Monopoly can even be educational.

Date Night

What could be more important than a date night with the one you love? Getting out of the house for a date night is always special, but sometimes, after the family begins to grow, a night out is not always in the budget. With a sheet, a candle, and some flowers in a vase, anyone can create a romantic setting to share with their date. Consider pulling out the best dishes to make it even more of a special moment. If you are feeling extra romantic, you could even string up some white lights above your table to set the mood.

The best advice I can give for a date night is to set one. Period. Whether it is once a week, every other week, or once a month, special time should always be set aside. We mark our calendar for all other kinds of events, so marking down a date night should be just as important.

Fun with Friends

Laughter that fills the air is a great way to find connection with the people you love. Game night for two or a fun night with friends can be a great way to bond and strengthen relationships. Who doesn't love a table filled with finger foods and delightful desserts? Put it on the calendar and start a fun new tradition with your favorite people. Fix a special treat or dress up your popcorn with chocolate and candy pieces. Anything so long as it's fun and out of the ordinary.

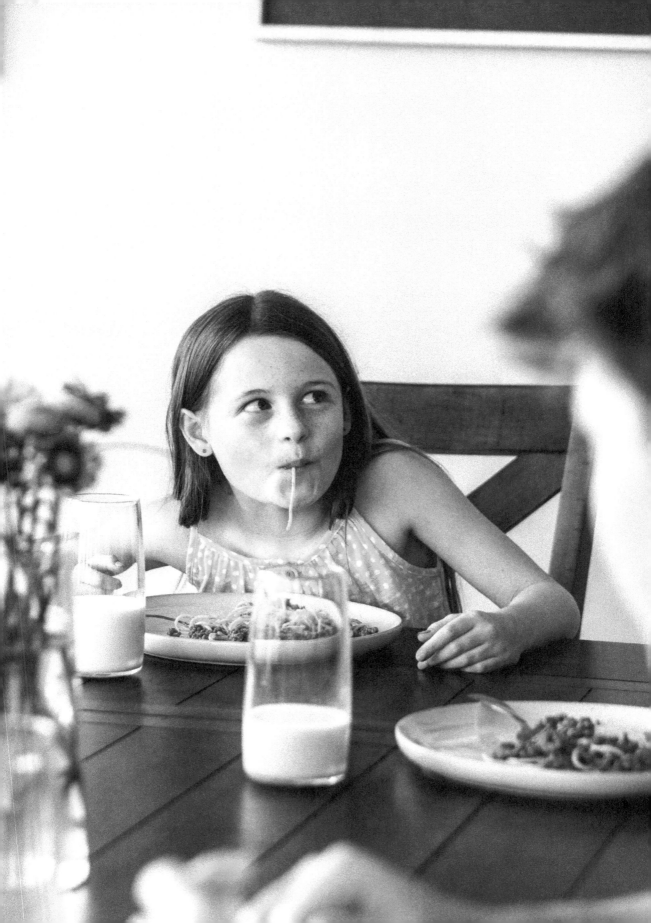

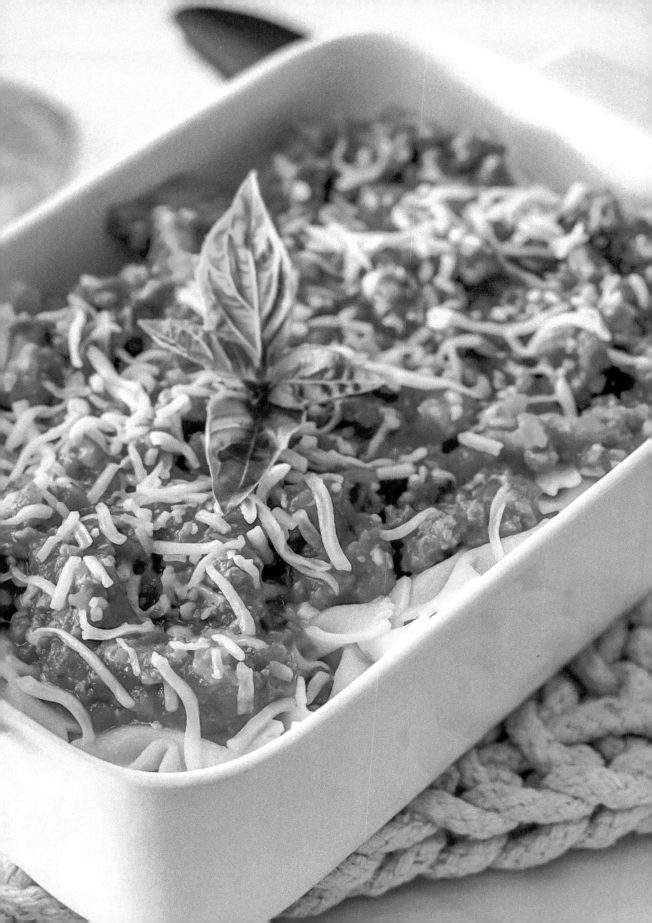

Easy Baked Pasta

Prep Time: 20 min. / **Cook Time:** 30 min. / **Serves:** 4

INGREDIENTS:

1 lb. lean ground beef
1 (24 oz.) jar pasta sauce of choice
1 (16 oz.) container low-fat cottage cheese
2.5 cups uncooked bow-tie pasta
1 Tbsp. chopped fresh basil
2 cups mozzarella cheese, divided

INSTRUCTIONS:

1) Preheat oven to 350°F.
2) In a medium skillet, cook ground beef until crumbled. Add sauce and stir in fresh basil.
3) Cook noodles according to package.
4) In a medium lightly sprayed casserole dish, add a layer of noodles to the bottom. Spread 3/4 cup sauce over noodles. Spread 3/4 cup cottage cheese over sauce. Sprinkle 1/2 cup mozzarella cheese followed by another scoop of sauce. Sprinkle remaining mozzarella cheese over top.
5) Bake for 25-30 minutes until melted and bubbly.

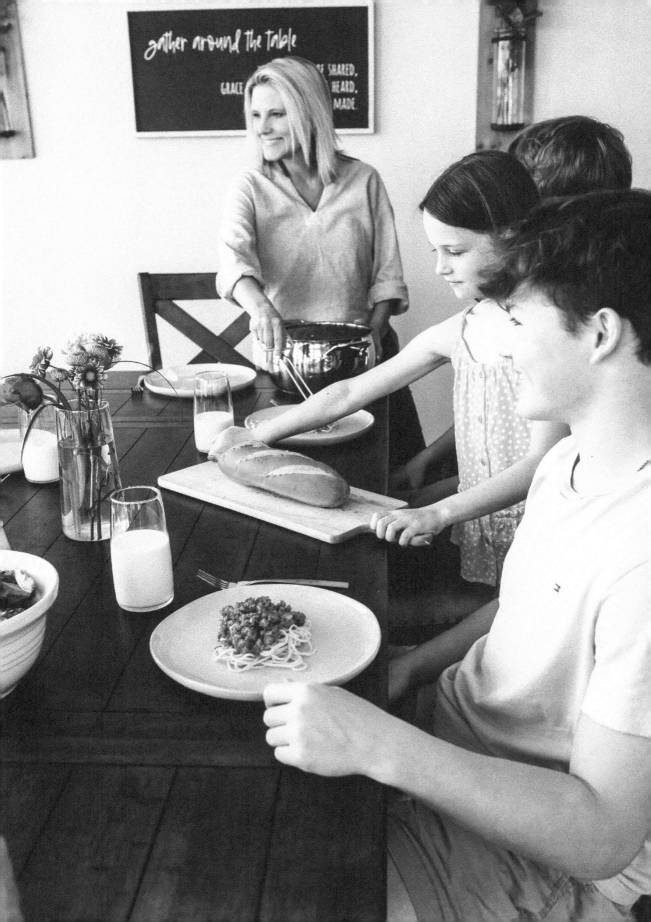

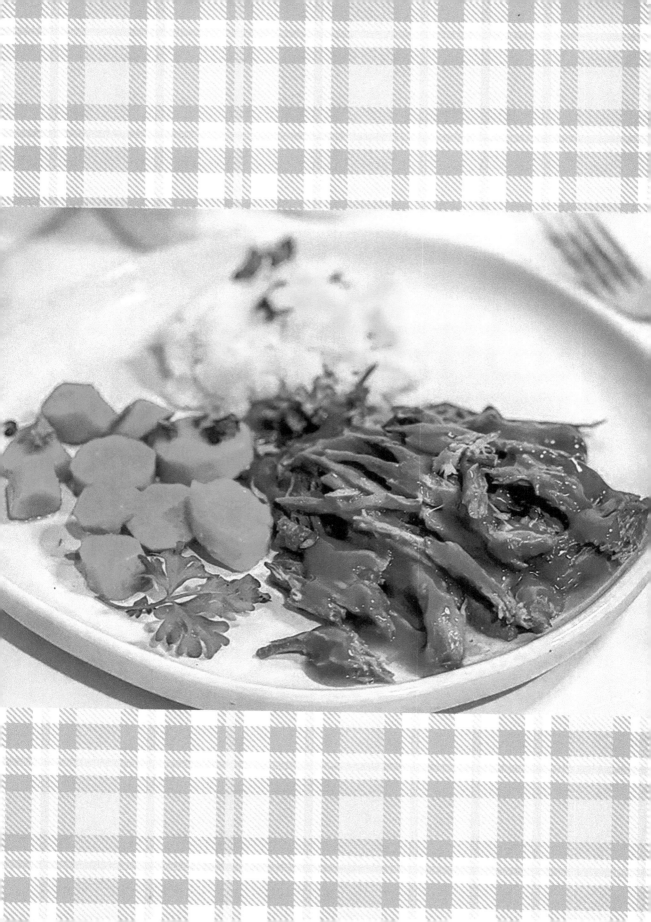

Simple Pot Roast

Prep Time: 5 min. / **Cook Time:** 8-10 hrs. / **Serves:** 4

Ingredients:

1 packet of dry Italian dressing mix
1 packet of dry ranch dressing mix
1 packet of brown gravy mix
1 1/2 cup of water
2-3 lbs. rump roast
3-4 carrots peeled and sliced into 1/2-inch rounds

Instructions:

1) Place roast in a crock pot. Sprinkle seasoning packets over top. Pour water around and over top roast.
2) Using a silicone basting brush, combine seasonings together and spread over roast. Place carrots around roast.
3) Cover and cook on high for 6-8 hours or on low for 8-10 hours.

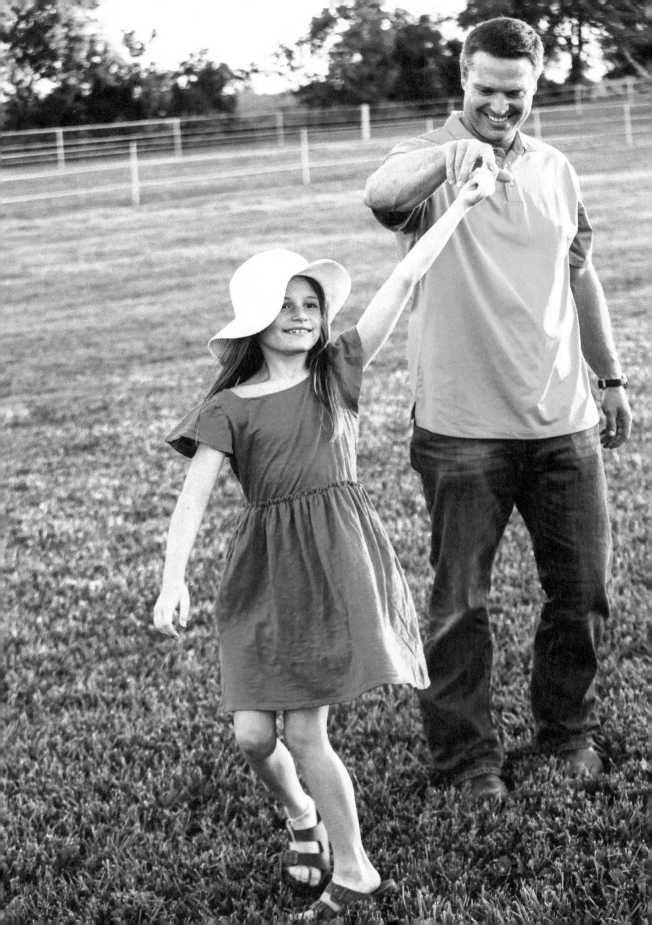

Sheet Pan Nachos

Prep Time: 10 min. / **Cook Time:** 10 min. / **Serves:** 4

INGREDIENTS:

1 lb. lean ground beef
1 pkg. low-sodium taco seasoning
Tortilla chips
1 (15 oz.) can black beans, drained and rinsed
1 cup prepared corn (frozen or canned)
1 tomato, diced
1 cup shredded cheddar cheese
Plain Greek yogurt, Jalapeño peppers, and cilantro for garnish

INSTRUCTIONS:

1) Preheat oven to 400°F.
2) Lightly spray baking sheet with non-stick spray.
3) Brown ground beef and add taco seasoning
4) Place tortilla chips in a single layer over baking sheet
5) Top with ground beef, beans, corn, and cheese. Bake for 5-7 minutes or until cheese is melted and bubbly.
6) Top with fresh cilantro, plain Greek yogurt, tomatoes, peppers, and any other desired toppings.

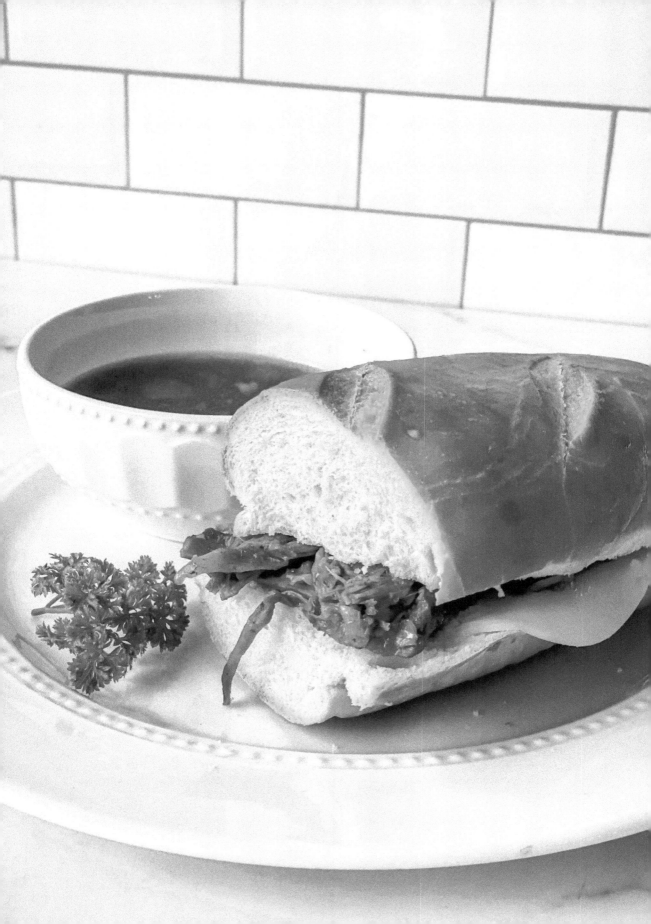

Slow Cooked French Dip

Prep Time: 10 min. / **Cook Time:** 6-8 hrs. / **Serves:** 4

INGREDIENTS:

3 lbs. beef chuck roast
1 (14.5 oz) can low-sodium beef broth
1 large onion, thinly sliced
1 Tbsp. Worcestershire sauce
1/2 pouch French onion soup mix
2 cloves garlic, minced
1 fresh rosemary sprig
Freshly ground black pepper
Hoagie rolls or French bread
4 cups cooked Jasmine rice

INSTRUCTIONS:

1) Brown all sides of chuck roast in a large skillet over medium heat.
2) Place all ingredients in a crock pot on low for 6-8 hours or on high 4-6 hours.
3) Shred beef with a fork.
4) Serve with rice or on hoagie rolls.

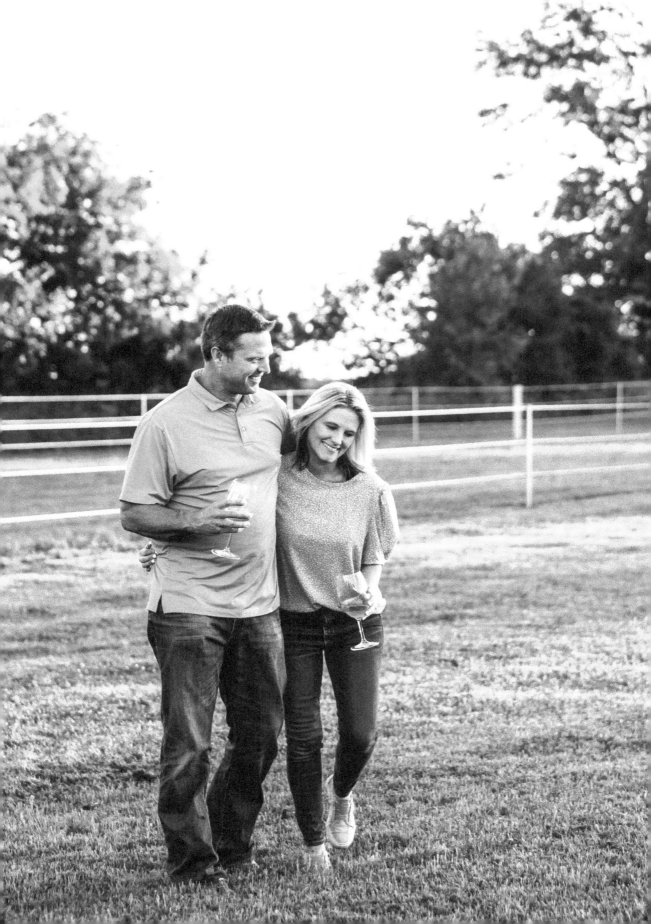

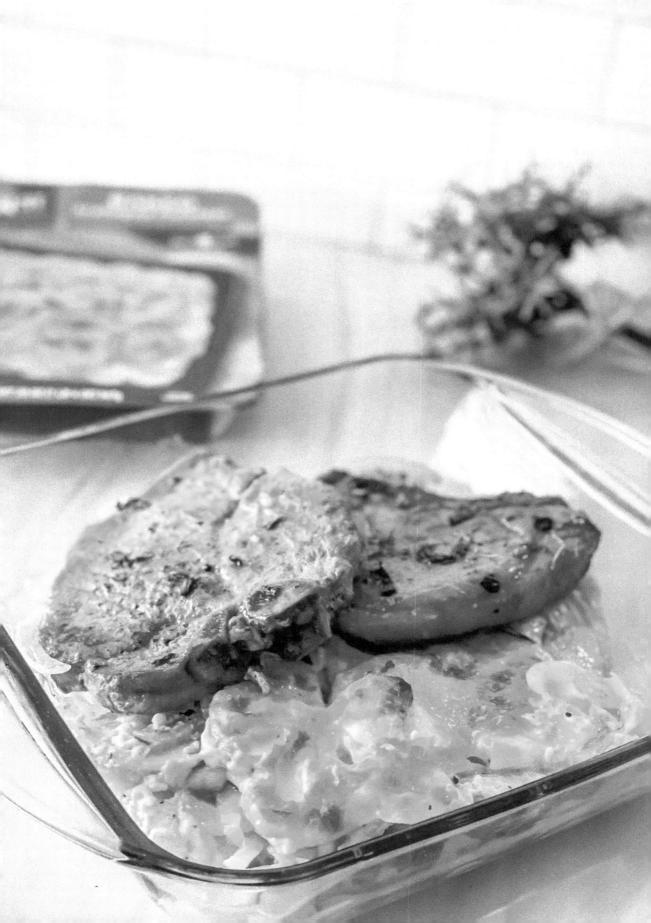

Pork Chops in a Garlic Butter Sauce

Prep Time: 5 min. / **Cook Time:** 12 min. / **Serves:** 2

Ingredients:

2 Tbsps. olive oil
2 bone-in pork chops
1 small yellow onion, chopped
2 Tbsps. butter
1 Tbsp. garlic, minced
Sea salt and cracked black pepper
1-2 fresh rosemary sprigs

Instructions:

1) In a large skillet, heat oil over medium heat until hot.
2) Pat dry and season pork chops with salt and pepper.
3) Sear pork chops 5-6 minutes per side or until brown. Transfer to a plate.
4) Add butter, garlic, rosemary, and onion to the skillet. Cook until garlic and onion are soft and translucent.
5) Place pork chops back into skillet. Spoon butter over pork chops, reduce heat to low, and cover.
6) Allow to simmer for 5 more minutes or until cooked through. Garnish with remaining rosemary.

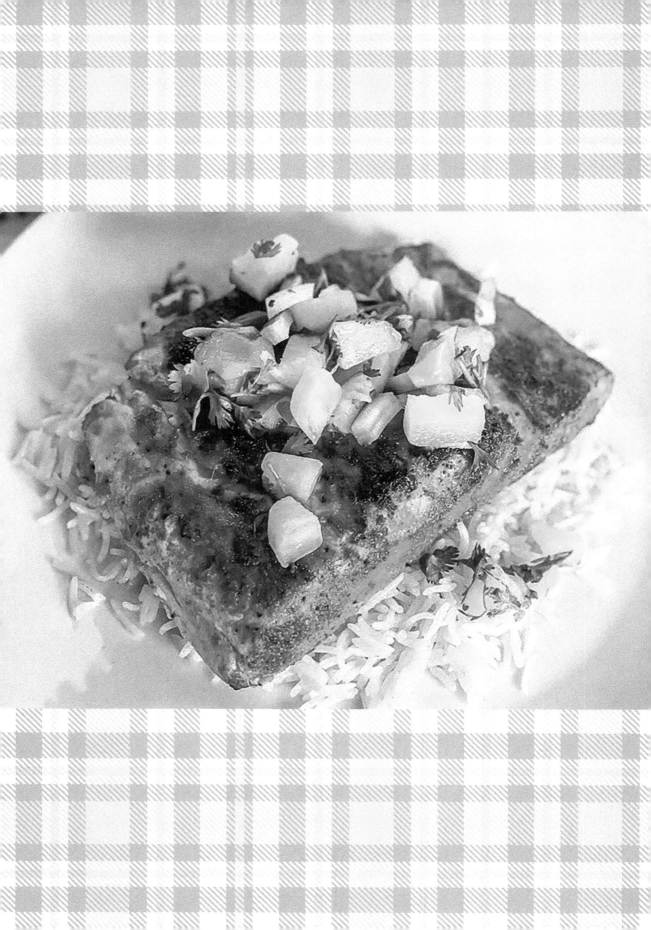

PAN-SEARED SALMON WITH PINEAPPLE SALSA

Prep Time: 20 min. / **Cook Time:** 10 min. / **Serves:** 2

INGREDIENTS FOR SALMON:

2 large salmon filets
1 tsp. chili powder
1 tsp. brown sugar (Swerve)
1/2 tsp. paprika
1/2 tsp. garlic, minced
1/2 tsp. onion powder
1/4 tsp. black pepper
1/2 tsp. sea salt

INGREDIENTS FOR PINEAPPLE SALSA

1/2 cup mango, diced small
1/2 cup pineapple, diced small
1/4 cup red onion, diced small
1 Tbsps. cilantro, finely chopped
Juice from a lime

INSTRUCTIONS FOR SALMON:

1) Combine all seasonings together in a small bowl and lay on a plate.
2) Gently pat-dry salmon filet and place in seasoning blend; fully coat side without the skin.
3) Heat a medium-sized skillet on high heat with olive oil. Reduce heat to medium and place salmon filets seasoned-side down.
4) Once you are done searing the salmon on the seasoned side, flip to sear skin-side down for an additional 6 minutes over medium heat. You may carefully remove the skin from the salmon at this time with a pair of tongs and sprinkle seasoning over top.
5) Once cooked all the way through, you can set aside while you make the pineapple mango salsa.

INSTRUCTIONS FOR PINEAPPLE SALSA:

1) Combine all ingredients together in a small bowl and squeeze juice of 1/2 lime over top.
2) Serve over rice and enjoy!

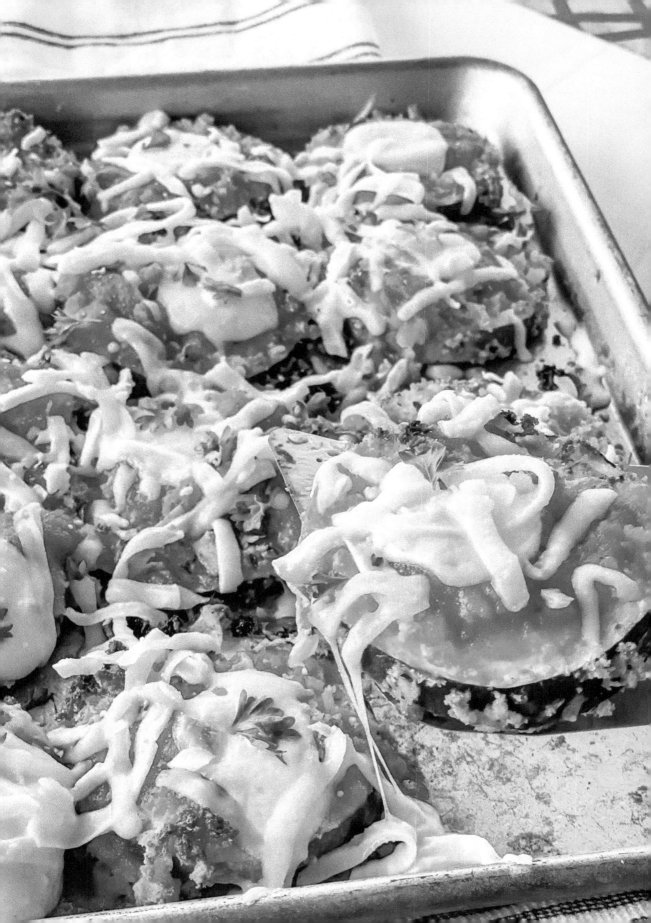

Zucchini Parmesan

Prep Time: 20 min. / **Cook Time:** 20 min. / **Serves:** 2

Ingredients:

1/2 cup breadcrumbs
1/3 cup Parmesan cheese, freshly grated
Salt and pepper, for taste
2 large eggs, beaten
1 medium zucchini, 1/4-inch sliced rounds
1/3 cup all-purpose flour
1/2 cup marinara sauce of choice
1/2 cup shredded mozzarella
1 Tbsp. fresh parsley, chopped
1 tsp. fresh oregano, chopped

Instructions:

1) Preheat the oven to 400°F.
2) Spray a rimmed baking sheet or shallow dish with non-stick spray.
3) In a medium bowl, combine breadcrumbs, fresh herbs, salt, and pepper.
4) Place beaten eggs in a small bowl and sprinkle flour on a plate.
5) Begin by coating zucchini rounds one by one in flour.
6) Drench zucchini in beaten egg, then coat each round with breadcrumbs.
7) Place breaded zucchini on a baking sheet in a single layer and bake for 18-20 minutes until golden brown.
8) Remove from the oven and set aside. Turn the oven to broil.
9) Add a spoonful of marinara over each zucchini round and top with mozzarella cheese.
10) Place back into the oven on broil for 2-3 minutes until melted.
11) Sprinkle with fresh parsley and serve.

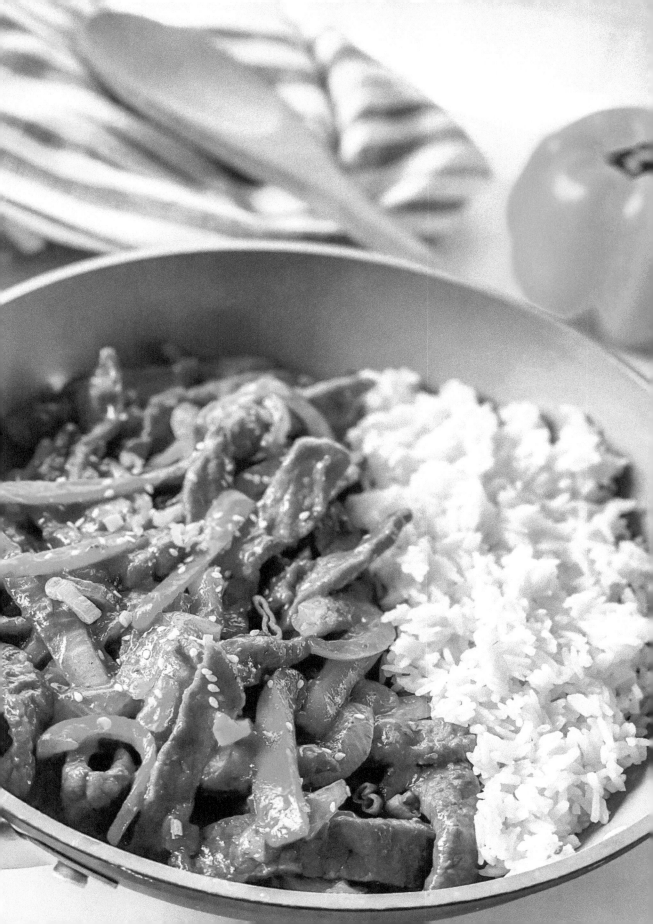

Pepper Steak and Onions

Prep Time: 10 min. / **Cook Time:** 5 min. / **Serves:** 2

Ingredients:

Eye of round steak, sliced thin
1 Tbsp. olive oil
1 yellow bell pepper, sliced thin
1 red bell pepper, sliced thin
1 small onion, sliced thin
1/4 cup liquid aminos (soy sauce)
1 tsp. red wine vinegar
2 Tbsps. honey
1 ½ Tbsps. cornstarch, dissolved in water
1 tsp. Sriracha
Green onion and sesame seeds to garnish
Salt and pepper, for taste

Instructions:

1) In a large skillet over medium heat, add oil.
2) Add steak strips and cook approximately 5 minutes until no longer pink.
3) Season with salt and pepper for taste.
4) Add vegetables and sauté for approximately 3-5 minutes.
5) Add liquid aminos, honey, red wine vinegar, sriracha, and corn starch. Cook until sauce thickens.

5

From Scrambled to Sunnyside

"If you look at the world, you'll be distressed. If you look within, you'll be depressed. If you look at God you'll be at rest." –**Corrie ten Boom**[33]

CRACKED BUT NOT BROKEN. I DON'T KNOW ABOUT YOU, but this title gives me so much hope for my life. No matter what comes my way, I can continue on. This is true for every one of us. Disruptions in our mental health will not go away by simply ignoring them. We need to do our part by recognizing the cracks we are experiencing and giving others time to recognize their own. As we identify these cracks, we will be able to develop ways to prevent them from making us feel broken.

No Shame in Asking for Help

According to NAMI, National Alliance of Mental Health, one in twenty-five U.S. adults experience serious mental illness. Fifty percent of all mental illnesses begin at age fourteen, and 75 percent by age twenty-four. The common warning signs of mental illness are as follows:[34]

- Feeling very sad or withdrawn for more than two weeks
- Trying to harm or end one's life or making plans to do so
- Severe, out-of-control, risk-taking behavior that causes harm to self or others
- Sudden overwhelming fear for no reason, sometimes with a racing heart, physical discomfort, or difficulty breathing
- Significant weight loss or gain
- Seeing, hearing, or believing things that aren't real*
- Excessive use of alcohol or drugs
- Drastic changes in mood, behavior, personality, or sleeping habits
- Extreme difficulty concentrating or staying still

- Intense worries or fears that get in the way of daily activities

While I understand that some people can experience levels of depression and anxiety without suffering from mental illness, I wanted to ensure these key factors were listed out. Any of the above bullet points which might plague you without relief could be a sign of a mental illness and should not be overlooked. Mental health is health. It is important to seek a professional to discuss these matters rather than assume they will eventually disappear on their own.

Bestselling author and pastor Levi Lusko spoke about his own lingering depression in his book, *Through the Eyes of a Lion*. In 2012, five days before Christmas, Levi and his wife lost their five-year-old daughter, Lenya, to an asthma attack. This experience pushed him toward professional help when the sadness continued to linger despite any efforts. It is important to realize seeking help does not make us weak. Speaking to counselors or being prescribed medication does not make us weak. These things are stepping stones to strengthen us.[35]

There is no shame in reaching out for help. While friends and family can provide excellent listening ears and advice, there are times when they may not be qualified to provide the right kind of help in some situations. Seeking help from a trained licensed professional can greatly improve your quality of life if you struggle with mental illness.

All the Way to the Root

Counselors aim to dig down to the root cause of the issue while also recognizing triggers that can arise and how to diffuse them. When we seek help for our mental health, it does not mean we are broken or damaged. Instead, it means we want to help ourselves for a better tomorrow. We deserve a quality of life that is peaceful and fulfilled. In order for that to happen, we must be willing to put in the time even when we don't want to.

Think of counseling like planting a garden. If we planted seeds in an unprepared field, the crop would not grow properly. Most of the seeds wouldn't penetrate the hard soil on their own, and the seeds who did would most likely be choked out by weeds before they could produce anything worth a harvest.

The same thing happens when pain and trauma are left alone. Most of us desire to be healthy and prosperous; we seek good things for ourselves and our families, yet we try to plant these seeds in an unprepared field. Unattended childhood trauma or rejection will lead to trust issues and the desire for acceptance. This can then lead to hanging around bad influences simply to gain approval.

Jumping from one relationship straight into another is usually a surefire way to see it fail. Why? Because the ground was not properly prepared. Let's look at it in the kitchen. You don't cook up spaghetti sauce, serve it to the family, and immediately start cooking something else in the pot, do you? No. The pot needs to be cleaned before starting something new otherwise there will be things from the old dish that will blend into the new dish.

Sometimes our lives need a light rinse with water and then we are ready to go. Other times, there is some deep cleaning with a whole lot of elbow grease to prepare us for the next thing in life. While counseling can benefit us in either situation, it is always in our court to admit when we need outside help.

Self-Evaluation

Each of us is different, and we deal with stress and the pressures of life in our own unique way. Many people have promoted their unique solutions through books, blogs, and other social platform posts. While we should not overlook how some cracks require professional help to overcome, we must also consider self-evaluation. There is so much value in pausing to connect with your own body. *Why am I reacting this way? Why am I feeling this way? How did that make me feel?* In addition to seeking professional help, there are many changes we can implement in our lives to help reduce the effects of the stresses we might be experiencing.

Self-evaluation can encompass many forms of activities from yoga to a bubble bath to painting to jogging. Each of us is different, so the way we reflect and recharge is also different. The most important part of this process is connecting with ourselves. Our eyes look outward and see everything going on in the world around us, which often means we neglect the world inside of us. We can have a major storm brewing inside yet never realize something is wrong until we yell at someone for something ridiculous.

Connecting with what's inside is an absolute must if we want to experience the sunny side of life. That is not to say things will be amazing, but the more we get in touch with ourselves, the more we will be able to exercise patience and self-control in situations we once were not able to. For more ways to reduce stress and calm the chaos in your life, see the resource section at the end of this book.

Life is difficult. It tosses us about unapologetically. While this leads to many cracks along the way, I hope you understand now that we don't have to accept brokenness. We can recognize our cracks and still find ourselves experiencing all of the sunny-side goodness this life has to offer. This kind of living is only possible when we choose to step out of the darkness and into the light—when we recognize it is okay not to be okay. Attempting to hide our cracks will only causes them to fester and grow. When we identify and address them, this is when we are able to grow. The process may vary from person to person, but each of us has the potential to enjoy life beyond our cracks.

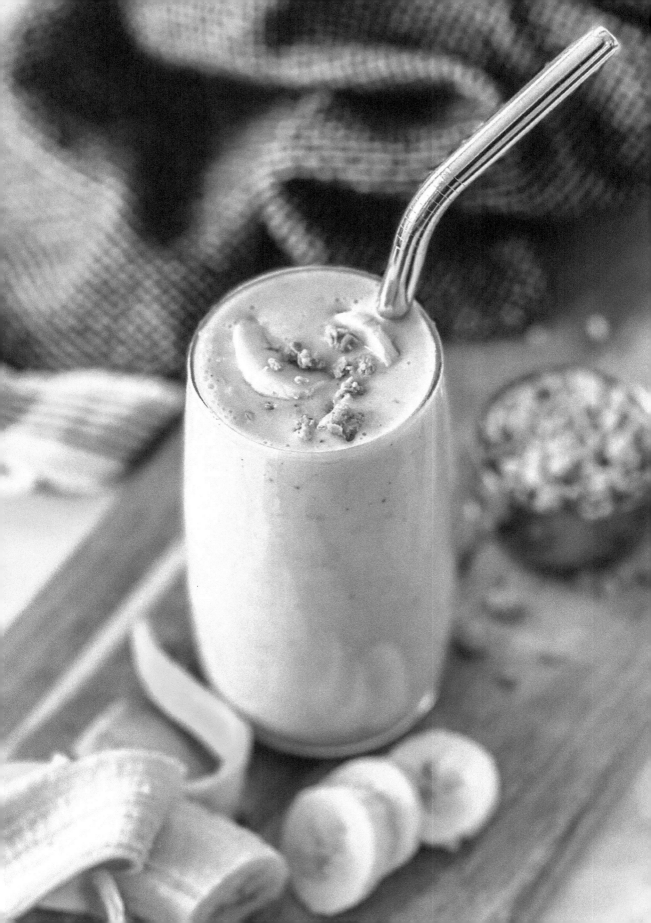

REFRESHING SMOOTHIES FOR THE SOUL

Self-care is likely one of the most important ways to move beyond the cracks in our lives. Incorporating a smoothie each day can be a great way to get a good portion of your nutrients. The health benefits of smoothies can be almost as diverse as their colors and textures. You can use smoothies for weight loss, fruit and vegetable intake, cleansing, a protein boost, and so much more. When mixing up your daily concoction, the sky is the limit on what you can add. For the best results, always stick to natural ingredients and avoid added sugars.

Peanut Butter Banana Smoothie

Prep Time: 5 min. / **Cook Time:** none / **Serves:** 1

INGREDIENTS:

2 frozen bananas
1/2 cup vanilla Greek yogurt
1 tsp. vanilla extract
1 tsp. honey
1 cup almond milk
1/2 cup natural creamy peanut butter
Dash of cinnamon over top

INSTRUCTIONS:

1) Combine all ingredients in a blender until smooth.

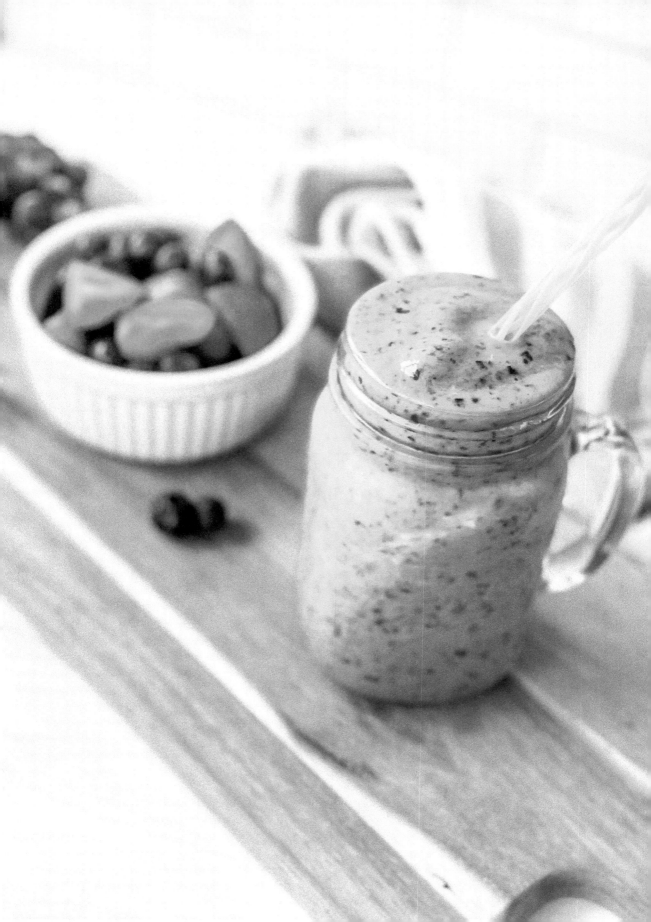

Berry Banana Smoothie

Prep Time: 5 min. / **Cook Time:** none / **Serves:** 1

INGREDIENTS:

1 cup fresh or frozen berries of choice
1/2 cup vanilla Greek yogurt
1 frozen banana
1/2 cup unsweetened almond milk
1 Tbsp. pure maple syrup
Fat free whip topping (optional)

INSTRUCTIONS:

1) Combine all ingredients in a blender until smooth.

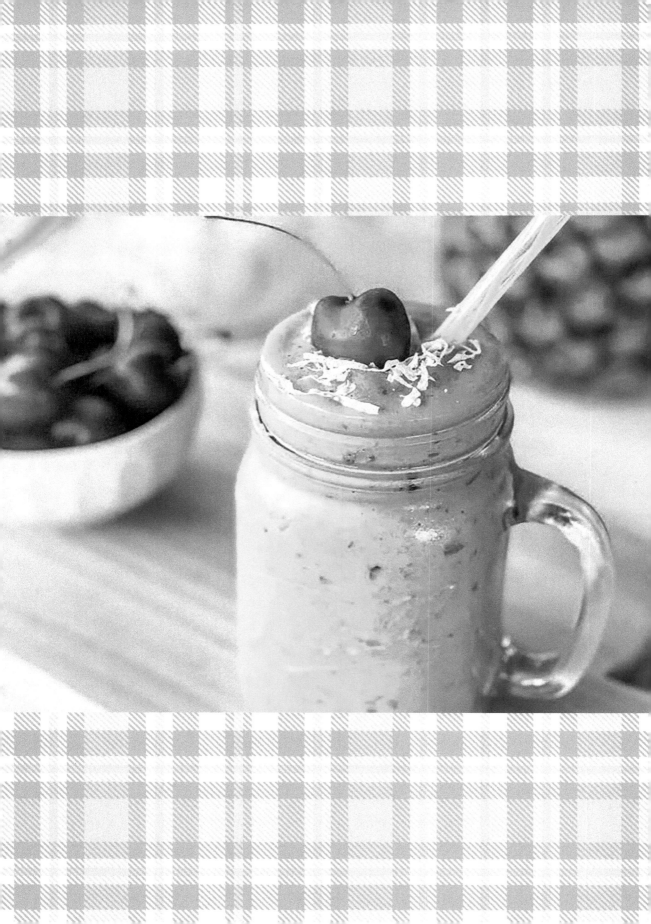

CHERRY PINEAPPLE SMOOTHIE

Prep Time: 5 min. / **Cook Time:** none / **Serves:** 1

INGREDIENTS:

1 cup plain Greek yogurt
3/4 cup frozen pitted cherries
3/4 cup frozen pineapple
3/5 cup coconut milk
Coconut flakes for garnish

INSTRUCTIONS:

1) Combine all ingredients in a blender until smooth.

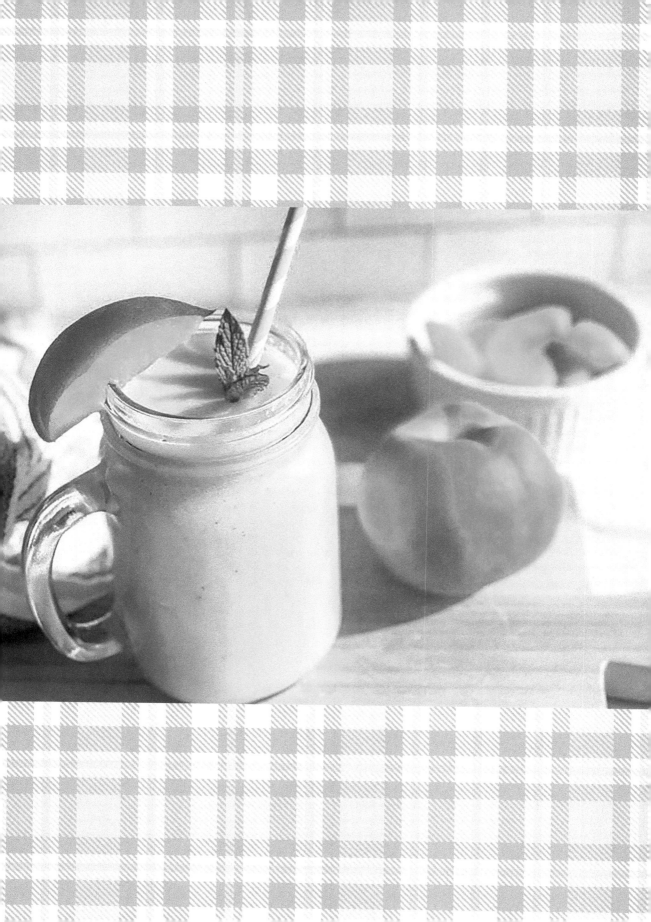

Peaches n' Cream Smoothie

Prep Time: 5 min. / **Cook Time:** none / **Serves:** 1

Ingredients:

1 frozen banana
1 cup frozen peaches, sliced
3/4 cup almond milk
1/3 cup cold water
1 Tbsp. honey
Pinch of nutmeg
Mint leaf to garnish

Instructions:

1) Combine all ingredients in a blender until smooth.

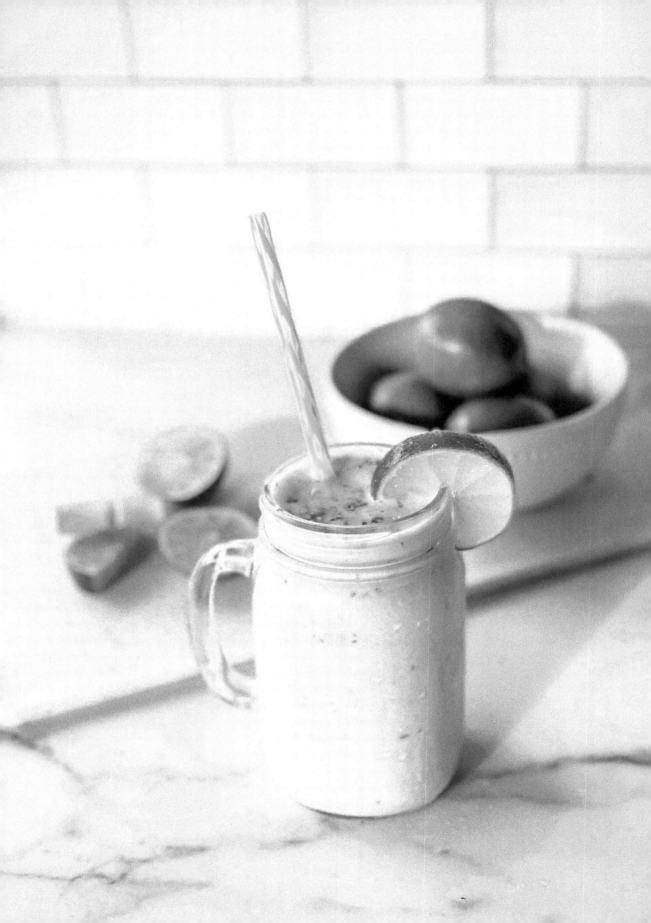

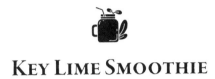

Key Lime Smoothie

Prep Time: 5 min. / **Cook Time:** none / **Serves:** 1

Ingredients:

1 ½ cup ice
1 cup Coco-Whip topping
1 lime, zested and squeezed
1/4 cup low-sugar orange juice
1/2 cup plain yogurt

Instructions:

1) Combine ingredients in a blender until smooth.

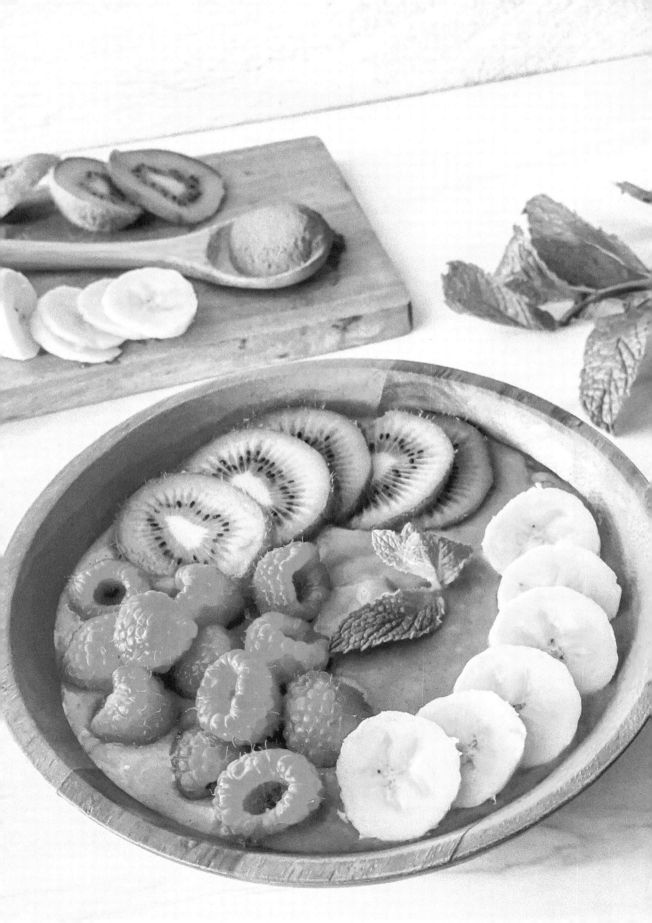

SUPERFOOD SMOOTHIE BOWL

Prep Time: 5 min. / **Cook Time:** none / **Serves:** 1

INGREDIENTS:

2 frozen bananas
1 cup frozen mango
1 tsp. Supergreens powder
1 scoop vanilla protein powder
1/4 cup unsweetened almond milk
Fresh sliced kiwi, banana and raspberries

INSTRUCTIONS:

1) Combine all ingredients in a blender until smooth and pour into a bowl.
2) Top with fresh kiwi, banana, and raspberries.

Techniques for Coping with Stress and Mental Illness

Yoga/Meditating

The great thing about yoga or meditation is the immediate pause it puts in our lives. Both require us to be quiet and listen. These are qualities that have faded within our busy society. It seems as if we are always on the move and there is always noise bombarding us. Taking a quiet moment allows us to listen to our body and figure out where the issues lie.

Positive Affirmations

Some people like listening to encouraging podcasts, others enjoy soothing, soft music. Most of the noise in our life tends to be negative and draining; switching over to something positive is a sure-fire way to pick up our spirit.

Finding a Hobby

Outdoor hikes, canoeing, mountain biking, painting, writing a book—there are so many hobbies a person can find. Most people find themselves with multiple hobbies, which spread across different seasons. Some might kayak rivers during the summer and work at a pottery wheel during the winter. Whatever the hobbies, they all point to one thing: taking time to enjoy the things we love to do. All work and no play will heighten the stress in our lives faster than anything else.

Take a Break

Speaking of all work and no play, the worst thing we can do for our mental health is refusing to take a break. Sometimes, this can be as simple as a thirty-minute lunch break. There will always be one more thing to do, one more person to help, and so on. If we do not take the time to breathe, we will find ourselves burnt out and overwhelmed. There are even times when a much longer break is needed. Maybe we need to take a vacation day to enjoy some of our hobbies or a week of vacation to reset and enjoy time with our loved ones. Once a day, once a week, once in a while, we need to give ourselves a break from the daily grind.

Physical Activity

There are many health benefits to physical activities. One of the best of those benefits is how it pumps up our endorphins. These are our brain's natural "feel-good" hormones. Whether it is swimming, walking, cycling, martial arts, boxing, aerobics class, or whatever your preference may be, physical activity is a great way to combat many of the things which drag us down.

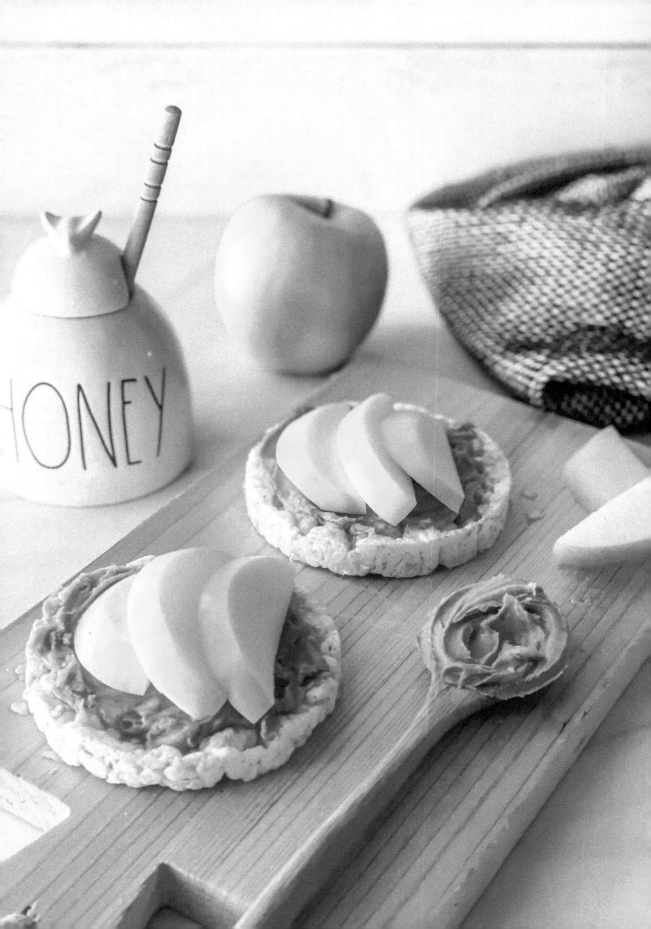

TREAT YOURSELF: SNACKS & DESSERTS

There's something to be said for treating yourself when times are tough. These simple snack recipes are delicious and nutritious!

Peanut Butter & Apple Rice Cakes

Prep Time: 5 min. / **Cook Time:** none / **Serves:** 2

INGREDIENTS:

1 Tbsp. all-natural peanut butter
1 apple of choice
2 unsalted rice cakes
1 tsp. honey

INSTRUCTIONS:

1) Spread a thin layer of peanut butter over each rice cake.
2) Top with apple slices and drizzle honey over top.

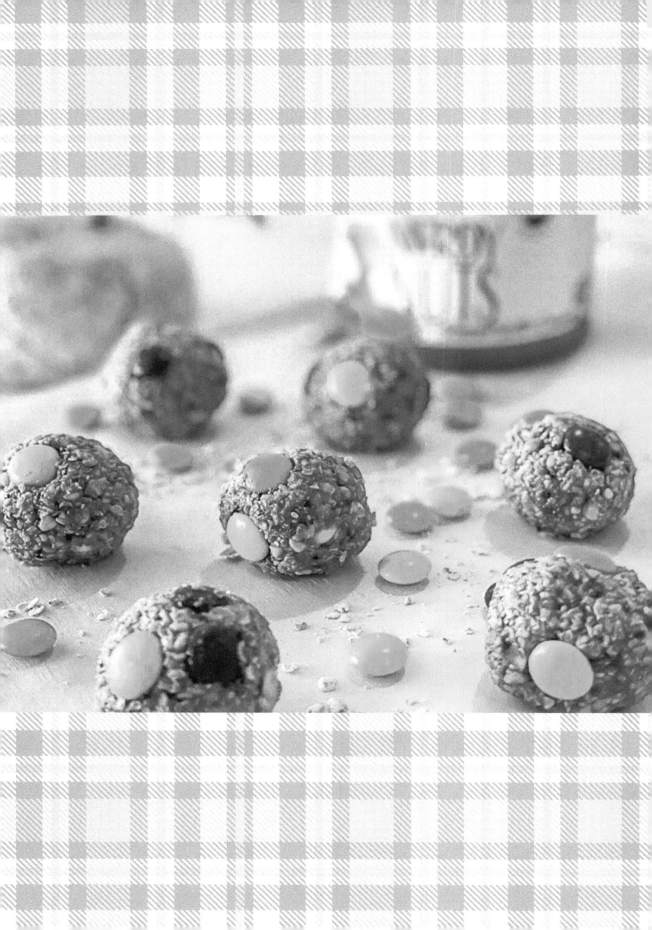

Peanut Butter Protein Balls

Prep Time: 30 min. / **Cook Time:** none / **Serves:** 2

Ingredients:

1 1/2 cups rolled oats
1 tsp. cinnamon
1 Tbsp. chia seeds
1/2 cup natural peanut butter
2 Tbsps. honey
2 Tbsps. maple syrup
Handful of Reese's pieces
Pinch of salt

Instructions:

1) Combine dry ingredients first.
2) Incorporate remaining ingredients into mixture and begin forming balls 1-inch in diameter.
3) Place on parchment paper in a covered container and let sit in the refrigerator approximately 30 minutes and serve.

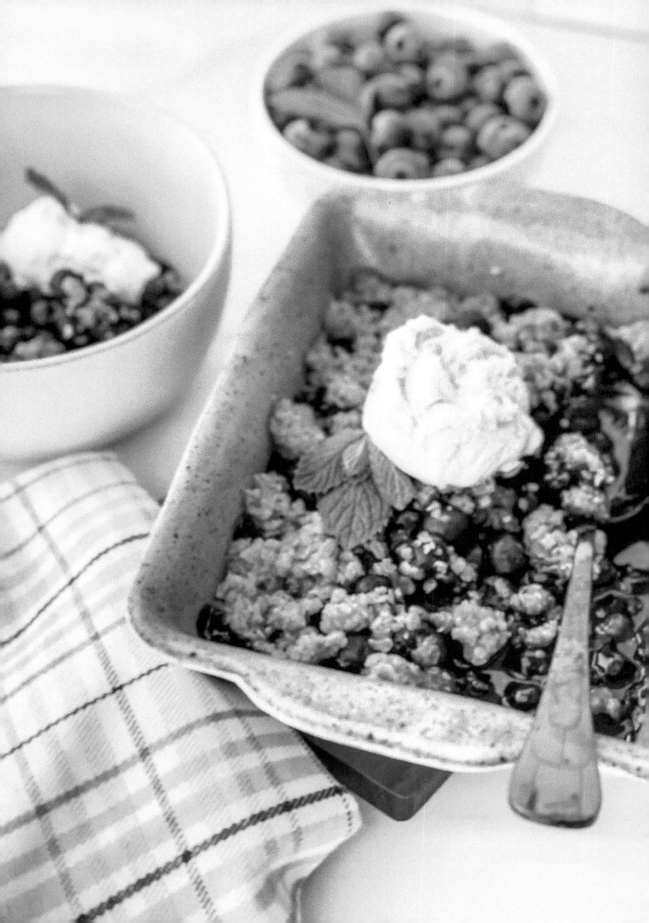

Easy Blueberry Crisp

Prep Time: 10 min. / **Cook Time:** 30 min. / **Serves:** 4

Ingredients for Filling:

2 1/2 cups fresh or frozen blueberries
1/2 tsp. vanilla extract
1/2 Tbsp. lemon juice
1 1/2 Tbsps. flour (all-purpose or white whole-wheat)
Pinch of sea salt
Whipped topping (optional)

Ingredients for Topping:

1/2 cup rolled oats
2 Tbsps. flour (all-purpose or white whole-wheat)
3 Tbsps. light brown sugar
Pinch of sea salt
3 Tbsps. softened butter, unsalted

Instructions:

1) Preheat the oven to 375ºF and spray a small 6x8-inch casserole dish with nonstick cooking spray.
2) Combine all of the ingredients for the filling in a large bowl and transfer to the baking dish. Set aside.
3) In a separate bowl, combine and prepare crumble topping.
4) Evenly spread topping over the berries.
5) Place in the oven and bake for 30 minutes.
6) Serve with whipped topping (optional).

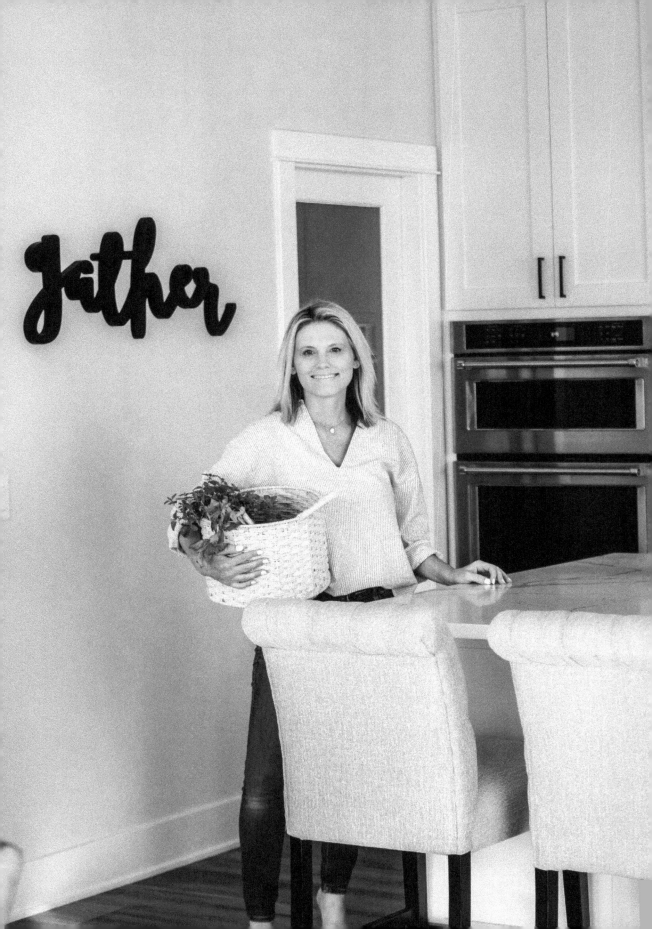

Authors Note

Thank you for joining me on this journey of finding hope through some of life's deepest cracks. I hope these words touched your soul the same way they touched mine while writing this. I hope you leave feeling lifted in some way, ready for a new tomorrow.

If you loved this book and have a minute to spare, I would really appreciate a short review or mention where you bought the book. Reviews from readers like you make a huge difference in helping new readers feel inspired the same way you have.

Thank you!

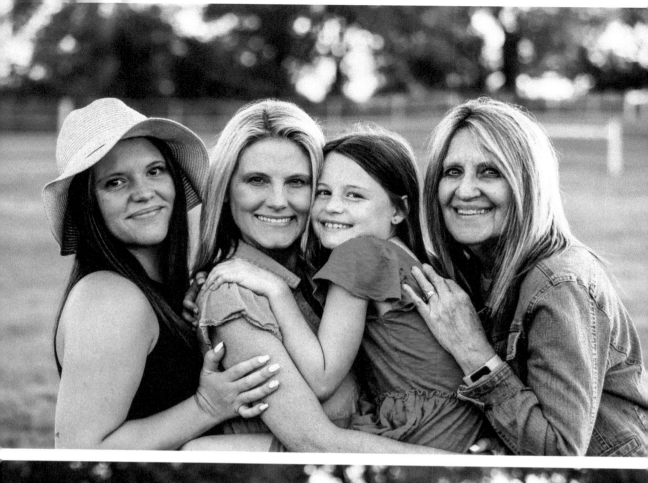
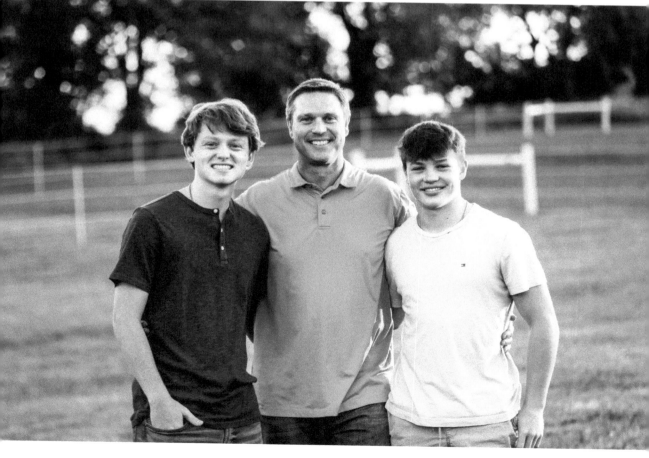

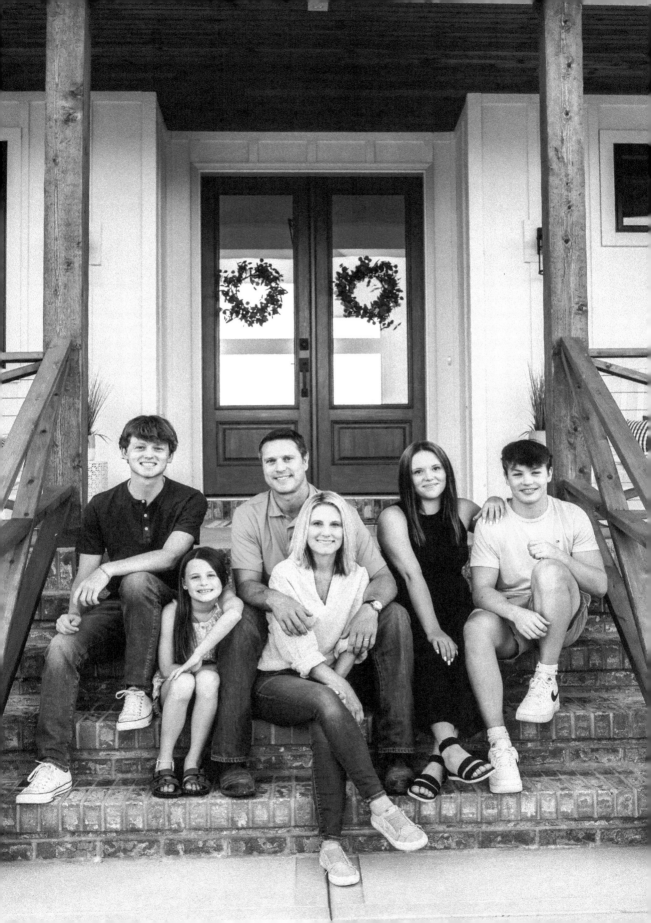

What To Do In a Crisis

D ISRUPTION TO OUR MENTAL HEALTH CAN LEAD MANY down a very dark path. If you or someone you know is in crisis, tell someone who can help right away:

- Call your doctor's office
- Call 911 for emergency services
- Go the nearest hospital emergency room
- Call the toll-free, 24-hour hotline of the National Suicide Prevention Lifeline at (800) 273-8255 to be connected to a trained counselor at a suicide crisis center nearest you

If you have a family member or friend in crisis, do not leave him or her alone. Try to get the person to seek help immediately. Stay in touch with them, check up on them often, and if necessary, ensure they get the help they need. In some instances, it may be necessary to request law enforcement to perform a well-check if they are avoiding communication with others.

Endnotes

1   Linda Poindexter Quotes, Quotable Quote, accessed June 22, 2022, https://www.goodreads.com/quotes/603958-one-small-crack-does-not-mean-that-you-are-broken

2. Shannon L. Alder Quotes, Quotable Quote, accessed June 22, 2022,https://www.goodreads.com/quotes/7085204-there-is-no-perfection-only-beautiful-versions-of-brokenness

3   Arthur Rubinstein Quotes, Quotable Quote, accessed June 22, 2022, https://www.goodreads.com/quotes/40996-of-course-there-is-no-formula-for-success-except-perhaps

4   Bryant McGill Quotes, Quotable Quote, Simple Reminders: Inspiration for Living Your Best Life accessed June 22, 2022, https://www.goodreads.com/quotes/1312228-rejection-is-merely-a-redirection-a-course-correction-to-your

5   Ed Sheeran, Twitter Post, accessed June 22, 2022, https://twitter .com/edsheeran/status/122630364886859776?lang=en

6   Thomas Curran and Andrew P. Hill, "Perfectionism Is Increasing, and That's Not Good News", accessed June 20.2022, https://hbr.org/2018/01/perfectionism-is-increasing-and-thats-not-good-news

7   "21 Egg Facts for World Egg Day 2021". Retrieved March 2022. https://www.val-co.com/21-fun-egg-facts-for-world-egg-day-2021/

8   Charles R. Swindoll, AZ Quotes, accessed June 20,2022,https://www.azquotes.com/quote/592690

9   Jodi Picoult Quotes, Quotable Quotes, Jodi Picoutl, House Rules, accessed June 20, 2022, https://www.goodreads.com/quotes/267103-rest-easy-real-mothers-the-very-fact-that-you-worry

10 https://www.lifeway.com/en/articles/surrounded-by-worry

11 Ed Rowell, "Learn to Drop the Worry Habbit", last modified January 1 2014, accessed June 22, 2022, https://www.goodreads.com/quotes/7946633-instead-of-worrying-about-what-you-cannot-control-shift-your

12 "The Best Instant Pot tips, tricks, and hacks". By Michael Bizzaco and Erika Rawes.March 26, 2021. Digital Trends. https://www.digitaltrends.com/home/instant-pot-tips-and-tricks/

13 "5 Mistakes Everyone Makes With Their Instant Pot". Cheryl S. Grant. Updated: Nov. 04, 2020. Taste of Home. https://www.tasteofhome.com/article/instant-pot-mistakes/

14 "18 (Seriously Useful) Instant Pot Tips, Tricks, And Hacks: Whether you're a proud new owner or you've been using an IP for years." Melissa Jameson. BuzzFeed. https://www.buzzfeed.com/melissaharrison/instant-pot-hacks-accessories

15 "Living So That Lesson Five: Let Your Light Shine So That [Giveaway!], Nov. 21, 2014, accessed June 22, 2022, https://wendyblight.com/2014/11/living-so-that-lesson-five-let-your-light-shine-so-that/

16 "Are you ready to address your suffering?", Joe Roller Counseling, accessed June 22, 2022, https://www.joerollercounseling.com/counseling-for-trauma

17. Richard Puz Quotes, The Carolinian, accessed June 22, 2022, https://www.goodreads.com/quotes/862483-death-leaves-a-heartache-no-one-can-heal-love-leaves.

18 Eskimo Proverb Quotes, Quotable Quote, accessed June 22,2022, https://www.goodreads.com/quotes/7086953-perhaps-they-are-not-stars-but-rather-openings-in-heaven

19 Beth Moore, AZ Quotes, accessed June 22,2022, https://www.azquotes.com/quote/809035

20 Timothy Leary Quotes, Quotable Quote, accessed June 22, 2022, https://www.goodreads.com/quotes/8510830-if-you-want-to-change-the-way-people-respond-to

21 Khalil Gibran, AZ quotes, accessed June 22, 2022, https://www.azquotes.com/quote/529713

22 Christine Caine, Unshakeable: 365 Devotions for Finding Unwavering Strength in God's Word (Michigan, Zondervan Publishing, 2017), 124

23 7 Promises from God to Remind Us: He Will Bring Good From the Storms in Our lives, Debbie McDaniel, Feb 02, 2017, accessed June 22, 2022, https://

www.ibelieve.com/faith/7-promises-to-remind-us-god-will-bring-good-from-the-storms-in-our-lives.html

24 5 Self-Love Languages, LINK, accessed June 22, 2022, https://www.linkbcit.ca/5-self-love-languages/

25 Shirley Chisholm, Brainy Quotes, accessed June 22, 2022, https://www.brainy-quote.com/quotes/shirley_chisholm_797104

26 Louisa Alcott/ Life Quotes, Mind Journal, accessed June 22.2022, https://the-mindsjournal.com/be-the-woman-who-fixes-another-womans-crown/

27 Lady Bird Johnson Quotes, Quotable Quote, accessed June 22, 2022, https://www.goodreads.com/quotes/10400005-encourage-and-support-your-kids-be-cause-children-are-apt-to

28 Charles M. Shultz quotes, accessed June 22, 2022, https://quotefancy.com/quote/998052/Charles-M-Schulz-In-life-it-s-not-where-you-go-it-s-who-you-travel-with

29 https://www.goodreads.com/quotes/13374-you-don-t-love-someone-because-they-re-perfect-you-love-them

30 Jodi Picoult Quotes, Quotable Quote, My Sister's Keeper, accessed June 22, 2022, https://instagramcircus.com/loving-family-quotes/

31 Michael J. Fox, Brain Quote, accessed June 22, 2022, https://www.brainyquote.com/quotes/michael_j_fox_189302

32 Retrieved March 2022 from Tarrant Area Food Bank Website. Article origi-nally posted August 26, 2020. https://tafb.org/blog/the-importance-of-fami-ly-meals-nb25/?gclid=CjwKCAjwrfCRBhAXEiwAnkmKmSennyUo-IAjWL-Ht0ZF-xno78vHvSVdRT99JEMGp3fyIzYWyjh2k7BoCRY0QAvD_BwE

33 Corrie ten Boom Quotes, Quotable Quote, accessed June 22, 2022, https://www.goodreads.com/quotes/32394-if-you-look-at-the-world-you-ll-be-distressed-if

34 "Less Than One-Third of Adults with Mental Illness Will Get Help in 2009" NAMI, Sept. 24,2009, accessed June 22, 2022, https://www.nami.org/Press-Media/Press-Releases/2009/Less-Than-One-Third-of-Adults-with-Mental-Illness

35 Levi Lusko, "Through the Eyes of a Lion: Facing Impossible Pain, Finding Incredible Power", (Thomas Nelson, Nashville, TN, 2015)

CPSIA information can be obtained
at www.ICGtesting.com
Printed in the USA
BVHW022331091122
651654BV00005B/18